Epidemiology of Sleep Disorders: Clinical Implications

Guest Editor

EDWARD O. BIXLER, PhD

SLEEP MEDICINE CLINICS

www.sleep.theclinics.com

March 2009 • Volume 4 • Number 1

SAUNDERS an imprint of ELSEVIER, Inc.

W.B. SAUNDERS COMPANY
A Division of Elsevier Inc.

1600 John F. Kennedy Boulevard • Suite 1800 • Philadelphia, PA 19103-2899

http://www.sleep.theclinics.com

SLEEP MEDICINE CLINICS Volume 4, Number 1
March 2009, ISSN 1556-407X, ISBN-13: 978-1-4377-0540-9, ISBN-10: 1-4377-0540-5

Editor: Sarah E. Barth
Developmental Editor: Donald Mumford

Sleep Medicine Clinics (ISSN 1556-407X) is published quarterly by Elsevier, 360 Park Avenue South, New York, NY 10010. Months of issue are March, June, September and December. Business and Editorial Office: 1600 John F. Kennedy Blvd., Ste. 1800, Philadelphia, PA 19103-2899. Accounting and Circulation Offices: 11830 Westline Industrial Drive, St. Louis, MO 63146. Periodicals postage paid at New York, NY, and additional mailing offices. Subscription prices are $150.00 per year (US individuals), $76.00 (US students), $339.00 (US institutions), $149.00 (Canadian individuals), $106.00 (Canadian students), $373.00 (Canadian institutions), $185.00 (foreign individuals), $106.00 (foreign students), and $373.00 (foreign institutions). Foreign air speed delivery is included in all *Clinics* subscription prices. All prices are subject to change without notice. **POSTMASTER:** Send change of address to *Sleep Medicine Clinics*, Elsevier, Periodicals Customer Service, 11830 Westline Industrial Drive, St. Louis, MO 63146. Customer Service (orders, claims, online, change of address): **Elsevier Periodicals Customer Service, 11830 Westline Industrial Drive, St. Louis, MO 63146. Tel: 1-800-654-2452 (U.S. and Canada); 314-453-7041 (outside U.S. and Canada). Fax: 314-453-5170. E-mail: journalscustomerservice-usa@elsevier.com (for print support); journalsonline-support-usa@elsevier.com (for online support).**

Reprints. For copies of 100 or more of articles in this publication, please contact the Commercial Reprints Department, Elsevier Inc., 360 Park Avenue South, New York, NY 10010-1710. Tel.: 212-633-3812; Fax: 212-462-1935; E-mail: reprints@elsevier.com.

Printed and bound by CPI Group (UK) Ltd, Croydon, CR0 4YY
Transferred to Digital Print 2012

GOAL STATEMENT

The goal of *Sleep Clinics of North America* is to keep practicing physicians up to date with current clinical practice by providing timely articles reviewing the state of the art in patient care.

ACCREDITATION

The *Sleep Clinics of North America* is planned and implemented in accordance with the Essential Areas and Policies of the Accreditation Council for Continuing Medical Education (ACCME) through the joint sponsorship of the University of Virginia School of Medicine and Elsevier. The University of Virginia School of Medicine is accredited by the ACCME to provide continuing medical education for physicians.

The University of Virginia School of Medicine designates this educational activity for a maximum of 15 *AMA PRA Category 1 Credits*™. Physicians should only claim credit commensurate with the extent of their participation in the activity.

The American Medical Association has determined that physicians not licensed in the US who participate in this CME activity are eligible for 15 *AMA PRA Category 1 Credits*™.

Credit can be earned by reading the text material, taking the CME examination online at http://www.theclinics.com/home/cme, and completing the evaluation. After taking the test, you will be required to review any and all incorrect answers. Following completion of the test and evaluation, your credit will be awarded and you may print your certificate.

FACULTY DISCLOSURE/CONFLICT OF INTEREST

The University of Virginia School of Medicine, as an ACCME accredited provider, endorses and strives to comply with the Accreditation Council for Continuing Medical Education (ACCME) Standards of Commercial Support, Commonwealth of Virginia statutes, University of Virginia policies and procedures, and associated federal and private regulations and guidelines on the need for disclosure and monitoring of proprietary and financial interests that may affect the scientific integrity and balance of content delivered in continuing medical education activities under our auspices.

The University of Virginia School of Medicine requires that all CME activities accredited through this institution be developed independently and be scientifically rigorous, balanced and objective in the presentation/discussion of its content, theories and practices.

All authors/editors participating in an accredited CME activity are expected to disclose to the readers relevant financial relationships with commercial entities occurring within the past 12 months (such as grants or research support, employee, consultant, stock holder, member of speakers bureau, etc.). The University of Virginia School of Medicine will employ appropriate mechanisms to resolve potential conflicts of interest to maintain the standards of fair and balanced education to the reader. Questions about specific strategies can be directed to the Office of Continuing Medical Education, University of Virginia School of Medicine, Charlottesville, Virginia.

The faculty and staff of the University of Virginia Office of Continuing Medical Education have no financial affiliations to disclose.

The authors/editors listed below have identified no professional or financial affiliations for themselves or their spouse/partner:
Rashmi Nisha Aurora, MD; Sarah Barth (Acquisitions Editor); Edward O. Bixler, PhD (Guest Editor); Cynthia Brown, MD (Test Author); Rohit Budhiraja, MD; Susan Calhoun, PhD; Julio Fernandez-Mendoza, PsyD; Anthony Kales, MD; Xian Li, MD, MS; Duanping Liao, MD, PhD; Jiahao Liu, MD; Susan Dickerson Mayes, PhD; Maurice M. Ohayon, MD, DSc, PhD; Sara Olavarrieta-Bernardino, PsyD; Slobodanka Pejovic, MD; Stuart F. Quan, MD; Sol Rodriguez-Colon, MS; Antonio Vela-Bueno, MD; Alexandros N. Vgontzas, MD; and Terry Young, PhD.

The authors/editors listed below have identified the following professional or financial affiliations for themselves or their spouse/partner:
Donald L. Bliwise, PhD serves on the Speakers Bureau for Takeda and Boehringer Ingelheim, and serves as a consultant and on the Advisory Committee/Board for Takeda.
Teofilo Lee-Chiong, Jr., MD (Consulting Editor) is an independent contractor for NIH, Restore, Respironics, Schwarz Pharma, and Takeda, and is a consultant for Elsevier.
Naresh M. Punjabi, MD, PhD serves as an industry funded research/investigator for Resmed Inc. and as a lecturer for CME syposia for Resmed Inc. and Respironics Inc.

Disclosure of Discussion of Non-FDA Approved Uses for Pharmaceutical Products and/or Medical Devices.
The University of Virginia School of Medicine, as an ACCME provider, requires that all faculty presenters identify and disclose any off-label uses for pharmaceutical and medical device products. The University of Virginia School of Medicine recommends that each physician fully review all the available data on new products or procedures prior to clinical use.

TO ENROLL

To enroll in the Sleep Clinics of North America Continuing Medical Education program, call customer service at 1-800-654-2452 or visit us online at http://www.theclinics.com/home/cme. The CME program is available to subscribers for an additional fee of $99.95.

Sleep Medicine Clinics

FORTHCOMING ISSUES

June 2009

Circadian Rhythms and Sleep
Kenneth P. Wright, Jr., PhD,
Guest Editor

September 2009

Polysomnography
Lawrence J. Epstein, MD,
Douglas Kirsch, MD,
Guest Editors

December 2009

Behavioral Sleep Medicine
Kenneth L. Lichstein, MD,
Guest Editor

RECENT ISSUES

December 2008

Respiratory Disorders and Sleep
Ulysses J. Magalang, MD, *Guest Editor*

September 2008

Neurologic Disorders and Sleep
Michael H. Silber, MBCHB, *Guest Editor*

June 2008

The Psychiatric Dimensions of Sleep Medicine
Karl Doghramji, MD, *Guest Editor*

March 2008

Sleep and Disorders of Sleep in Women
Helen S. Driver, PhD, RPSGT, DABSM,
Guest Editor

THE CLINICS ARE NOW AVAILABLE ONLINE!

Access your subscription at:
www.theclinics.com

Contributors

CONSULTING EDITOR

TEOFILO LEE-CHIONG, Jr., MD
Head, Division of Sleep Medicine, National Jewish
Health; Associate Professor of Medicine,
University of Colorado Denver School of Medicine,
Denver, Colorado

GUEST EDITOR

EDWARD O. BIXLER, PhD
Professor; Director of the Sleep Research and
Treatment Center, Penn State College of
Medicine, Hershey, Pennsylvania

AUTHORS

R. NISHA AURORA, MD
Assistant Professor of Medicine, Division of
Pulmonary, Critical Care, and Sleep Medicine,
Mount Sinai School of Medicine, New York,
New York

EDWARD O. BIXLER, PhD
Professor; Director of the Sleep Research and
Treatment Center, Penn State College of
Medicine, Hershey, Pennsylvania

DONALD L. BLIWISE, PhD
Professor of Neurology, Program in Sleep, Aging
and Chronobiology, Emory University School of
Medicine, Wesley Woods Health Center, Atlanta,
Georgia

ROHIT BUDHIRAJA, MD
Assistant Professor of Medicine, Section of
Pulmonary and Critical Care Medicine, Southern
Arizona VA Healthcare System and University of
Arizona College of Medicine, Tucson,
Arizona

SUSAN CALHOUN, PhD
Assistant Professor; Senior Research Associate,
Department of Psychiatry, Sleep Research and
Treatment Center, Penn State College of
Medicine, Hershey, Pennsylvania

JULIO FERNANDEZ-MENDOZA, PsyD
Human Sleep and Applied Chronobiology
Laboratory, Department of Psychiatry,
Universidad Autonoma de Madrid, Madrid,
Spain

ANTHONY KALES, MD
Professor Emeritus and Founding Chairman,
Department of Psychiatry, Penn State
University College of Medicine, Hershey,
Pennsylvania

XIAN LI, MD, MS
Department of Public Health Sciences,
Pennsylvania State University College
of Medicine, Hershey, Pennsylvania

DUANPING LIAO, MD, PhD
Department of Public Health Sciences,
Pennsylvania State University College
of Medicine, Hershey, Pennsylvania

JIAHAO LIU, MD
Department of Public Health Sciences,
Pennsylvania State University College
of Medicine, Hershey, Pennsylvania

SUSAN DICKERSON MAYES, PhD
Professor and Chief Psychologist, Department of Psychiatry, Milton S. Hershey Medical Center, Penn State College of Medicine, Hershey, Pennsylvania

MAURICE M. OHAYON, MD, DSc, PhD
Professor, Department of Psychiatry and Behavioral Sciences, School of Medicine, Stanford University, Stanford; Director, Stanford Sleep Epidemiology Research Center (SSERC), School of Medicine, Stanford University, Palo Alto, California

SARA OLAVARRIETA-BERNARDINO, PsyD
Human Sleep and Applied Chronobiology Laboratory, Department of Psychiatry, Universidad Autonoma de Madrid, Madrid, Spain

SLOBODANKA PEJOVIC, MD
Department of Psychiatry, Sleep Research and Treatment Center, Penn State College of Medicine, Hershey, Pennsylvania

NARESH M. PUNJABI, MD, PhD
Associate Professor of Medicine, Division of Pulmonary and Critical Care Medicine, Johns Hopkins University School of Medicine, Baltimore, Maryland

STUART F. QUAN, MD
Professor Emeritus of Medicine, Department of Medicine, Arizona Respiratory Center, University of Arizona College of Medicine, Tucson, Arizona; Visiting Professor of Medicine, Division of Sleep Medicine, Brigham and Women's Hospital, Harvard Medical School, Boston, Massachusetts

SOL RODRIGUEZ-COLON, MS
Department of Public Health Sciences, Pennsylvania State University College of Medicine, Hershey, Pennsylvania

ANTONIO VELA-BUENO, MD
Human Sleep and Applied Chronobiology Laboratory, Department of Psychiatry, Universidad Autonoma de Madrid, Madrid, Spain

ALEXANDROS N. VGONTZAS, MD
Professor and Endowed Chair in Sleep Disorders Medicine, Department of Psychiatry, Sleep Research and Treatment Center, Penn State College of Medicine, Hershey, Pennsylvania

TERRY YOUNG, PhD
Professor of Epidemiology, Department of Population Health Sciences, School of Medicine and Public Health, University of Wisconsin-Madison, Madison, Wisconsin

Contents

> The mechanisms for sleep-disordered breathing (SDB) in children are complex and
> share many of the etiologic risk factors with adults. Professionals who evaluate and
> treat children with SDB should be cognizant of comorbid risk factors associated with
> this disorder. Cardiovascular risk is a primary risk factor for SDB in children as in
> adults. Waist circumference and BMI are the consistent independent risk factors
> across several thresholds of severity of SDB. This finding suggests that, in children
> as in adults, metabolic and inflammatory factors may be an important mechanism in
> the development of SDB, implying that adenotonsillectomy may not always be the
> best first line treatment. Nasal abnormalities (eg, chronic sinusitis/rhinitis) were sig-
> nificant risk factors in children with milder SDB, suggesting that the evaluation and
> treatment of these abnormalities might be beneficial for this category of patients.
> Future research is indicated to confirm these findings, especially in children with
> moderate to severe SDB.

> Sleep-disordered breathing (SDB) is increasingly recognized as an important clinical
> problem in children; however, the clinical, anatomic, and physiologic correlates of
> SDB have not been studied extensively in a general population sample using poly-
> somnography to document the presence of SDB. The Tucson Children's Assess-
> ment of Sleep Apnea Study is a longitudinal cohort study of 503 Caucasian and
> Hispanic children aged 6 to 12 years old who underwent polysomnography and neu-
> rocognitive testing at the time of recruitment. Subsets of the cohort had additional
> MR imaging and pulmonary physiologic testing. Initial cross-sectional analyses indi-
> cate that SDB is associated with behavioral abnormalities, hypertension, learning
> problems, and clinical symptoms such as snoring and excessive daytime sleepi-
> ness. Future follow-up of the cohort will assess the impact of SDB on subsequent
> childhood development.

> Comparative analysis of parent-reported sleep problems in clinical and typical chil-
> dren shows that (1) children with anxiety or depression sleep more than children with

autism, ADHD-combined type, ADHD-inattentive type, acquired brain injury, and typical development; (2) children with autism have more sleep problems than children in the other diagnostic groups; (3) children with ADHD-inattentive type have the fewest sleep problems but have more daytime sleepiness than typical controls; (4) children with ADHD-combined type have more sleep problems than controls; (5) controls and children with ADHD-combined type have the least daytime sleepiness, and (6) children with brain injury have sleep problems scores in the midrange compared with all other groups.

Foreword

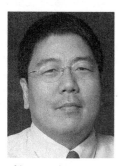

Teofilo Lee-Chiong, Jr., MD
Consulting Editor

Epidemiology is one of man's earliest achievements. As a science, it is second only to elementary mathematics—as humans learned how to count, distinguish, and classify people and their individual attributes, they were undertaking a task analogous to today's epidemiological processes.

The science of epidemiology had its foundations in rudimentary classification systems, which, in turn, became standardized as epidemiology evolved. It is this bi-directional relationship that provides both their individual strengths as well as perceived limitations. Ambiguous definitions of terms and indistinct delineations of relevant features always characterize any emerging scientific discipline, including sleep medicine. Thus, what were assumed to be valid historical, clinical, or laboratory parameters that our earlier classification systems were based upon had to undergo revisions to reflect the expanding understanding of sleep disorders. Comparisons between new epidemiological findings and historical census must take into account changes in terminology and nosology over time. Finally, epidemiologists should always consider cultural influences in the perception of behavior: what one society bans as deviant may be accepted in another time or place as individual idiosyncrasy.

It has been argued that nosological standardization must not only be assured among diverse studies but also for those that cross differing time periods. The latter is especially true for longitudinal studies that span decades. However, this viewpoint is potentially deceptive since classification systems evolve alongside progress in science. What is insomnia? Should its presence rely strictly on precise polysomnographic or actigraphic parameters, such as sleep onset latency, sleep efficiency, total sleep time, or wake time after sleep onset? Conversely, should it be defined based primarily on a person's complaints of disturbed or nonrestorative sleep? Are epidemiological data based on subjective descriptions (such as in the case of restless legs syndrome) less accurate than those that involve objective measures, including polysomnography for periodic limb movements during sleep? Are subjective measures of sleepiness (eg, Epworth sleepiness scale) truly reproducible, or do the inestimable biased effects of primacy, saliency, and recency make suspect their validity? Regarding the normal threshold for apnea-hypopnea indices across ages, from infancy to late adulthood, a single value is not applicable for all these population groups. Even the best analytical methods would be inadequate to correct for improper selection of measuring tools; as the latter are refined, becoming more sensitive or specific or both, do they nullify earlier studies, and if so, thwart attempts at comparison?

Herein lies a central scientific conundrum: in changing terminology and nosologic platforms, where does one start and when does one end? Epidemiological conclusions suffer at both extremes of frequency, ie, too frequent a change in nosology creates data incompatibility, and not frequent enough a change decays the conclusions into irrelevancy.

What then is the true worth of epidemiology? Are epidemiologists simply historians who record the events that transpire along the continuum of time, or are they more akin to artists who capture a single moment of time in paint, ink, or photographic paper? Neither, in any way, is fully able to define the present nor offer an assured perspective of the future. For some, it is enough to be

Sleep Med Clin 4 (2009) xi–xii
doi:10.1016/j.jsmc.2009.01.013
1556-407X/09/$ – see front matter

sleep.theclinics.com

aware that obstructive sleep apnea is as common as diabetes, without knowing the prevalence of each. Many know that obstructive sleep apnea is more common in men than in women; much fewer understand how these data were collected—nor care to know. Does an understanding of this gender difference in prevalence, therefore, play any major role in the selection of diagnosis and management approaches to suspected apnea in any specific individual? One has to distinguish between association and causation, ie, two events occurring together in time may be temporally correlated without one affecting the other.

Lastly, epidemiological exercises have been justified by arguing that their data have been utilized to determine proper allocation of scarce resources based on the relative prevalence of each medical disorder. But does this assumption hold true when one considers the widely divergent proportion of investments in time, personnel, and money for human immunodeficiency virus (HIV)

research compared to that for parasitic infections, such as malaria? Epidemiology will never replace agenda—personal or otherwise.

Humans will forever collect data and classify them—nevertheless, there are simply too much data to collect, from too many sources, and too little time and resources to do so. Men and women, therefore, will continue to gather data, as we have done in this issue of *Sleep Medicine Clinics*, aware that their task will never be complete.

Teofilo Lee-Chiong, Jr., MD
Division of Sleep Medicine
National Jewish Health
University of Colorado Denver School of Medicine,
1400 Jackson Street
Room J221
Denver, CO 60206, USA

E-mail address:
Lee-ChiongT@NJC.ORG (T. Lee-Chiong)

Preface

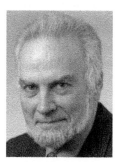

Edward O. Bixler, PhD
Guest Editor

Epidemiology is the study of distribution and determinants (risk factors) of risk for a disease in populations, and it is critical to the understanding of normal sleep patterns, as well as the distribution of and the risk for sleep disorders. It is considered a cornerstone of public health research and provides a quantitative foundation for public health policy, as well as a basis for preventative medicine and public health. From a historical perspective, Hippocrates is considered by some to be the father of epidemiology, as he described diseases according to place (endemic) and diseases focused in time (epidemic). A major focus of epidemiology is the minimization of bias. Most research methodologies share many of these types of bias (eg, internal and external validity). However, epidemiologic research pays particular attention to generalization and sampling issues. The increased sample size of most epidemiologic studies can increase the precision and the generalizability of the findings. In terms of sampling, many epidemiologic studies are based on volunteer samples while others obtain a truly representative sample. This latter strategy reduces the risk of selection bias, enhances generalizability, and improves the precision of the prevalence estimates. Thus, many modern epidemiologic studies have strived to obtain a truly representative sample.

Epidemiologic methodologies have contributed a great deal to our current understanding of normal sleep, as well as sleep disorders. The articles in this issue of *Sleep Medicine Clinics* are the outcome of a meeting held in Hershey, Pennsylvania, in November 2007 when representatives of the major epidemiologic cohorts within sleep were invited to participate. The intent was to bring together these various cohorts in order to share

common threads of findings and identify areas of disagreement requiring further study. This issue is organized by age of the subjects, beginning with children and concluding with adults. The initial article, by Dr. Bixler and colleagues, assesses the validity of some of the commonly used diagnostic criteria and etiologic risk factors for sleep-disordered breathing (SDB) based on a representative sample of elementary school children aged 5 to 12 years. The second article by Drs. Budhiraja and Quan describes the major results from the well established TuCASA child cohort, which was based on a sample of 6 to 12-year-old white and Hispanic children. The third review by Dr. Mayes and colleagues assesses the association of reported sleep problems with various childhood disorders based on a large clinical and community sample of children. In the following article, Dr. Liao, a cardiovascular epidemiologist, and his coauthors describes the association between autonomic balance in terms of heart rate variability and SDB based on a secondary analysis of the Penn State Child Cohort. The remaining six articles report on epidemiologic research involving adults. The review by Dr. Young describes her representative sample based on state employees aged 30 to 60 years, with four follow-up evaluations over 16 years. The next article is based on older adults: Drs. Punjabi and Aurora review the cardiovascular and non-cardiovascular consequences of SDB based on the largest multicenter cohort (subjects were recruited from several existing cardiovascular cohorts). The next review by Dr. Bliwise addresses the issue of the age dependence of SDB, based on the follow-up of one of the earliest established SDB cohorts. The following article is by Dr. Vgontzas and colleagues and evaluates

Sleep Med Clin 4 (2009) xiii–xiv
doi:10.1016/j.jsmc.2009.01.011

sleep.theclinics.com

the confounding effects of other sleep complaints and stress on the report of sleep duration independent of obesity based on the Penn State Cohort, which was a representative sample of the community between the ages of 20 and 100 years. The next review by Dr. Vela-Bueno and coauthors explores the sleep patterns reported by a large sample of college students. In the final article, Dr. Ohayon assesses the longitudinal association between insomnia and psychiatric disorders, organic diseases, and pain in a representative sample of the United States.

In closing, I want to thank all of the authors for taking time out of their busy schedules to contribute to this project. The list of authors was based on the participants in our original meeting. There were some investigators who were not able to attend this meeting or did attend but were not able to submit a manuscript. I gratefully want to thank Sarah Barth of Elsevier for her tenacious efforts in seeing this project through to its final form. I would also like to thank the Sleep Research and Treatment Center staff who made all of our data collection possible, and especially my longtime colleague and friend Dr. Vgontzas. Finally, I want to thank my mentor Dr. Kales, who taught me about the importance of testing hypotheses based on quality data, and most of all for his pioneering efforts in the establishment of the field of sleep medicine.

Edward O. Bixler, PhD
Department of Psychiatry MC:H073
Sleep Research and Treatment Center
Penn State College of Medicine
500 University Drive
Hershey, PA 17033

E-mail address:
ebixler@hmc.psu.edu (E.O. Bixler)

Commentary

Anthony Kales, MD

First, and foremost, I wish to pay tribute to my colleague of 39 years, Dr. Bixler. He has played a major role in our Sleep Research and Treatment Center: leading the conduct of a number of original, highly clinically relevant epidemiologic studies of sleep disorders and their physical and mental health correlates; assisting capably in our UCLA/Penn State series of studies that systematically assessed all major sleep disorders using the bio-psychosocial and behavioral model; and being primarily responsible for the successful transfer of our sleep laboratory from UCLA to Penn State in 1971 and skillfully directing it to the present time.

As Dr. Bixler has pointed out in his preface, epidemiologic studies provide us with not only important information on the prevalence of various disorders, but also on their correlates. Subsequent studies can help to delineate the role of the correlates, ie, causal, consequential, or comorbid. In our Los Angeles Metropolitan Area Survey (LAMAS) study,[1] we showed the high prevalence of sleep difficulty in the Los Angeles area, with the highest prevalence among women and with old age and reports of emotional difficulties. In our subsequent series of studies examining the bio-psychobehavioral correlates of subjects with a primary complaint of chronic insomnia,[2–5] as well as Healey's study of good and poor sleepers,[6] we delineated the role of mental and physical health correlates identified in the LAMAS study. We showed that predisposing mental and physical factors in childhood, and mental health problems in adulthood, mediated by poor coping mechanisms, when combined with increases in stressful life events, produce insomnia. The insomnia becomes chronic; that is, it is reinforced, maintained, and perpetuated through a vicious 24-hour cycle of mental distress, emotional hyperarousal,[5] physiological hyperarousal,[7] and conditioning factors, such as performance anxiety and fear of sleeplessness (Internalization Hypothesis).[2,3]

More recently, studies by our Penn State group, led by Dr. Vgontzas, have added to our original findings that chronic insomniacs are emotionally hyper-aroused throughout the day and night by their demonstrating that chronic insomniacs are physiologically hyper-aroused on a 24-hour basis.[8,9] These studies have shown that in chronic insomniacs, cortisol secretion is elevated throughout the day and night, and that cortisol activity relates positively to the degree of objective sleep disturbance. In this issue, the critical association of psychological factors with sleep disturbance is highlighted by the findings of Dr. Vgontzas and his colleagues: obese subjects with sleep complaints experienced significantly higher levels of emotional distress compared to those obese subjects without sleep complaints. As we found with our prior studies of subjects with a primary complaint of chronic insomnia, all eight clinical Minnesota Multiphasic Personality Inventory (MMPI) scales were significantly elevated.[2,3] It would be interesting to determine if the MMPI code patterns for these obese subjects with sleep complaints would fall into several distinct homogeneous code patterns indicating the primacy of psychological factors in their sleep disturbance, as was the case with our chronic insomniacs,[2,3] or if code patterns are heterogeneous and, thus, secondary to or a consequence of obesity and comorbid medical conditions, as is the case in various medical illnesses including sleep apnea[10] and narcolepsy/cataplexy.[11]

Ohayon demonstrates that insomnia, psychiatric disorders, organic diseases, and pain are closely interrelated. While the present intriguing data used major depressive disorder as a critical marker, it needs to be emphasized that in our studies, dysthymic depression together with obsessive-compulsive personality disorder or trait were the most prevalent diagnoses, by far, with only 4% of these chronic insomniacs having a principal diagnosis of major depressive disorder.[4]

Dr. Mayes stresses the importance of screening for sleep problems in children, especially with autism and Attention Deficit Hyperactivity Disorder-Combined Type (ADHD-C). Importantly, she points out that more than 50% of parents of children with autism report a sleep disturbance in their children, and that autistic children with sleep problems have more autistic symptoms relating to social and affective problems. Several papers relate to various aspects of sleep apnea in children and highlight various issues, including developmental

Sleep Med Clin 4 (2009) xv–xvi
doi:10.1016/j.jsmc.2009.01.010

factors, etiologic factors, and cardiovascular risk. Bixler and colleagues discuss the risk for elevated blood pressure and for neuropsychological impairment and suggest that in children, as is the case in adults, metabolic and inflammatory factors may be an important mechanism in the development of sleep-disordered breathing (SDB). In a related study of the Penn State Child Cohort, Dr. Liao and colleagues observed significant SDB-related and obesity-related impairment of cardiac autonomic modulation in children and stress the need for long-term studies assessing the cardiovascular risk for these findings. Budhiraja and Quans's findings suggest that obesity and SDB are associated with increased behavioral morbidity and learning impairment.

Dr. Young discusses the enormous societal burden of SDB and the additional concern that the prevalence will rise significantly along with the worldwide epidemic of obesity. For the near future, she believes continuous positive airway pressure (CPAP) holds the most hope for reducing the total societal burden of SDB. However, for CPAP to have a significant impact on the large numbers of patients with SDB, I believe much better diagnosis of the condition and much higher rates of compliance for the prescribed CPAP treatment are needed. For this to occur, physicians will need to be much more aware of the marked secondary psychological distress (denial and depression) that patients endure as a consequence of SDB[10] and utilize appropriate psychobehavioral educational measures. Further, looking at the total picture of sleep apnea as one part of the metabolic syndrome, appropriate treatment would have to include weight reduction, exercise, and sleep hygiene measures. Today, we rely almost solely on unidimensional therapy, ie, CPAP. I believe strongly that if physicians apply a multidimensional treatment mode to the metabolic syndrome and explain to patients the considerable morbidity and mortality of this condition, there will not only be greater compliance for CPAP treatment of SDB but also for the weight reduction and exercise needed for the effective management of the overall metabolic syndrome.

Dr. Vela-Bueno and his colleagues provide clinically relevant information and recommendations for prevention and coping with sleep disturbances in the transition period from adolescence to young adulthood. They apply and extend the general recommendations for sleep hygiene to this age group and emphasize regularity of sleep-wakefulness schedule; obtaining an adequate amount of sleep; napping properly (with supportive scientific evidence); avoiding "social jet lag;" minimizing arousing pre-bedtime activity; and avoiding sleep-disrupting substances.

Anthony Kales, MD
Department of Psychiatry
Penn State University College of Medicine
MB073 Psychiatry
Hershey, PA 17033

REFERENCES

1. Bixler EO, Kales A, Soldatos CR, et al. Prevalence of sleep disorders in the Los Angeles metropolitan area. Am J Psychiatry 1979;136:1257–62.
2. Kales A, Caldwell AB, Preston TA, et al. Personality patterns in insomnia: theoretical implications. Arch Gen Psychiatry 1976;33:1128–34.
3. Kales A, Caldwell AB, Soldatos CR, et al. Biopsychobehavioral correlates of insomnia. II: pattern specificity and consistency with the Minnesota Multiphasic Personality Inventory. Psychosom Med 1983; 45:341–56.
4. Tan T-L, Kales JD, Kales A, et al. Biopsychobehavioral correlates of insomnia, IV: diagnoses based on DSM-III. Am J Psychiatry 1984;141:357–62.
5. Kales JD, Kales A, Bixler EO, et al. Biopsychobehavioral correlates of insomnia V: clinical characteristics and behavioral correlates. Am J Psychiatry 1984;141:1371–6.
6. Healey ES, Kales A, Monroe LJ, et al. Onset of insomnia: role of life-stress events. Psychosom Med 1981;43:439–51.
7. Monroe LJ. Psychological and physiological differences between good and poor sleepers. J Abnorm Psychol 1967;72:255–64.
8. Vgontzas AN, Bixler EO, Lin H-M, et al. Chronic insomnia is associated with nyctohemeral activation of the hypothalamic-pituitary-adrenal axis: clinical implications. J Clin Endocrinol Metab 2001;86: 3787–94.
9. Vgontzas AN, Tsigios C, Bixler EO, et al. Chronic insomnia and activity of the stress system: a preliminary study. J Psychosom Res 1998;45:21–31.
10. Kales A, Caldwell AB, Cadieux RJ, et al. Severe obstructive sleep apnea – II: associated psychopathology and psychosocial consequences. J Chronic Dis 1985;38:427–34.
11. Kales A, Soldatos CR, Bixler EO, et al. Narcolepsy-cataplexy II: psychosocial consequences and associated psychopathology. Arch Gen Psychiatry 1982; 39:169–71.

The Penn State Child Cohort: Diagnostic Criteria and Possible Etiologic Factors of Sleep Apnea Based on Objective Clinical Outcomes

Edward O. Bixler, PhD*, Alexandros N. Vgontzas, MD, Susan Calhoun, PhD

KEYWORDS

- Apnea • Children • Epidemiology • Hypopnea
- Polysomnogram
- Sleep-disordered breathing

The criterion used for the diagnosis of sleep-disordered breathing (SDB) in adults has been reasonably well established against objective clinical outcomes. In children, however, the evaluation of diagnostic criteria against an objective clinical outcome has been limited. The majority of the available data have been based on clinical observation and relatively small samples. Limited population data have been available that have addressed this general issue.[1,2] The focus of the initial development of the Penn State Child Cohort (PSCC) was to establish a representative random sample of children aged 5–12 years of age. The initial goal was to assess various diagnostic criteria commonly used in relation to clinical morbidity. The two most obvious outcomes were blood pressure and neurocognitive impairment. Based on the optimal diagnostic criteria we further assessed a large set of potential risk factors for SDB in this cohort. This article reviews the basic methodology and the primary results of the initial cross-sectional data obtained from this cohort.

METHODS AND PROCEDURES
Basic Study Design

This study was designed as a two-phase study with the first phase collecting general information from the parents about their child's sleep and behavioral patterns.[3,4] The second phase collected more detailed data in our General Clinical Research Center (GCRC) on a stratified sample randomly selected from the first phase. The study was reviewed and approved by our Institutional Review Board as well as the GCRC review board.

In the first phase, elementary schools (K–5) were selected each year so that approximately 1500 students were enrolled. A questionnaire developed by Stradling[5] to be completed by a parent was sent home with every child in the elementary school. Over the course of five years, we sent home 7312 questionnaires and 5740 were returned for a response rate of 78.5%. In the second phase of this study, each year 200 children were selected from the questionnaires that were returned that year. Stratifying by grade, gender,

This article was supported by NIH grants: R01 HL63772, M01 RR010732, and C06 RR016499.

Department of Psychiatry, Sleep Research and Treatment Center, Penn State College of Medicine, H073, 500 University Drive, Hershey, PA 17033, USA

* Corresponding author.

E-mail address: ebixler@hmc.psu.edu (E.O. Bixler).

and risk for SDB (based on the parent's response to the initial questionnaire) we randomly selected children from each stratum in order to maintain representativeness of the original sample. The final sample included 700 children who completed a polysomnography (PSG) recording for a response rate of 70.0%. We observed no significant difference between the subjects who completed the PSG recording with those who were selected but did not complete the PSG recording.

Laboratory Polysomnography

For the sleep evaluation all subjects in the presence of a parent spent one night in sound-attenuated, temperature- and light-controlled rooms in our GCRC. The child's sleep was continuously monitored for nine hours with a four-channel electroencephalogram, a two-channel electro-oculogram, and a single-channel electromyogram. The sleep records were subsequently scored independently according to standardized criteria.[6] Respiratory airflow was monitored throughout the night by use of thermocouple at the nose and mouth, and nasal pressure and respiratory effort was measured with thoracic and abdominal strain gauges. We obtained an objective estimate of snoring during the PSG by monitoring breathing sounds with a microphone attached to the throat as well as a separate room microphone. All night, hemoglobin–oxygen saturation (SaO_2) was obtained from the finger.

An obstructive apnea was defined as a cessation of airflow with a minimum duration of 5 seconds and an out-of-phase strain gauge movement. A hypopnea was defined as a reduction of airflow of approximately 50% with an associated decrease in oxygen saturation (SaO_2) of at least 3% or an associated arousal. Based on these data an apnea index (AI) [apneas/hour of sleep] and an apnea/hypopnea index (AHI) [(apneas + hypopneas)/hour of sleep] were calculated.

Physical Examination

The physical examination, which was completed in the evening prior to the PSG, included height, weight, waist and neck measurement, blood pressure, a visual evaluation of the nose and throat by an ENT specialist, and an evaluation of respiratory function by a pediatric pulmonologist. Blood pressure was measured in the seated position using an automated system with appropriately sized cuffs. The mean of the final two of three blood pressure measurements were used for the analysis. Height was measured in centimeters using a stadiometer and weight was assessed in kilograms. In the standing position the waist was measured in

centimeters at the top of the iliac crest and the neck at the corticothyroid membrane.

Neuropsychologic Assessment

All children underwent a 2.5-hour neuropsychologic evaluation administered by a trained psychometrist prior to their overnight stay in the sleep laboratory at approximately the same time each afternoon. The following tests in the neuropsychologic battery were chosen in order to assess intelligence, and key neuropsychologic functions including: attention; executive functioning; memory; processing speed; mental flexibility; verbal fluency; and visual–motor skill.

Wechsler Abbreviated Scales of Intelligence (WASI) consists of four subtests corresponding to the same subtests on the *Wechsler Intelligence Scale for Children*, namely, WISC-IV (Block Design, Matrix Reasoning, Vocabulary, and Similarities) with a correlation of 0.87 with WISC-III Full Scale IQ in the general population.[7]

Gordon Diagnostic System (GDS) is a continuous performance test that has significant agreement with other measures of attention, including behavior rating scales, standardized observations, performance tests, and diagnoses of ADHD.[8]

WISC-III Digit Span is used as a measure of attention and working memory,[9] and in studies of children with ADHD it is the lowest of the WISC-III verbal subtest mean scores[10,11] and significantly lower than comparison children.[10]

Developmental Test of Visual-Motor Integration (VMI) measures visual–motor skills and is used to assess children with neurologic disorders, such as ADHD and autism.[12]

The *WISC-III Coding* subtest has demonstrated sensitivity to neuropsychologic impairment and is low in children with neurologic disorders such as ADHD, autism, and learning disability.[10–13]

Animal Naming Test (ANT) is widely used as a measure of verbal fluency (specifically retrieval from semantic memory) in child neuropsychologic assessment batteries.[14]

California Verbal Learning Test (CVLT) measures verbal learning and memory and is sensitive to neurologic impairment[15] and severity of brain injury.[16]

Stroop Color and Word Test–Children's Version (Stroop) is a measure of executive functioning[17] in terms of ability to shift cognitive inhibition and ability to inhibit an overlearned dominant response in favor of an unusual one.[18]

Wisconsin Card Sorting Test–64-Card Version (WCST-64) is a shortened version of the well-regarded 128-card version that measures executive functioning and has been shown to be sensitive to frontal lobe dysfunction in children.[19]

ASSOCIATION BETWEEN BLOOD PRESSURE AND SLEEP-DISORDERED BREATHING IN CHILDREN
Blood Pressure is Not Associated with Apnea Indices

Current clinical standards use two different definitions to diagnose SDB, one based on AI and the other on AHI. Neither of these criteria has been assessed based on a relevant objective clinical outcome. To address this issue we first assessed the association of SDB, based on these two definitions, and blood pressure, a clinical outcome frequently associated with SDB in adults.[3] The association of AI with blood pressure was assessed by comparing those with AI < 1 and subjects with AI > 1 and AI > 2. There was no significant association between AI and blood pressure. We did observe a significant increase in blood pressure associated with AHI thresholds ranging from AHI ≥ 1 to AHI ≥ 5 compared with AHI < 1 (**Fig. 1**). Because we did not observe a significant association between AI and blood pressure, all of our further analyses were based on the AHI.

Blood Pressure is Not Associated with Rapid-Eye Movement Apnea/Hypopnea Indices

It has been reported that SDB in children, in contrast to adults, is a REM-related disease.[20] To assess this hypothesis we first evaluated the association between REM and non-REM AHI

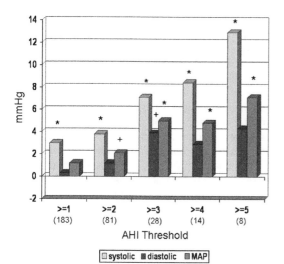

Fig. 1. The increase in blood pressure (systolic, diastolic, and MAP) for AHI thresholds ranging from 1–5 compared with those with an AHI < 1. Significance based on ANCOVA controlling for age, gender, and height percentile. *P <.01. +P <.05. N is presented in parentheses.

with the severity of the overall AHI.[3] The correlation between the REM AHI and the overall AHI was markedly less than the correlation between the non-REM AHI and the overall AHI (REM R^2 = 0.112, non-REM R^2 = 0.947). The average AHI observed in our sample during REM sleep was 1.12 ± 0.07 (median 0.48, interquartile range [IQR] 1.54) compared with 0.74 ± 0.07 (median 0.18, IQR 0.78) during non-REM sleep (signed rank test P <.001), which supports the hypothesis that more AHI occurred in REM than in non-REM in children.

To assess the relative clinical significance among these AHI groups we first divided our subjects into three groups based on AHI < 1, 1 ≤ AHI < 5, and AHI ≥ 5. We assessed the differences between these three groups using analysis of covariance (ANCOVA) adjusted for sampling weight, age, minority, sex, BMI percentile, sleep efficiency, snoring, and percentage of REM sleep. In terms of the relationship with blood pressure, the NREM AHI was significantly associated with elevated systolic blood pressure (P <.0002) whereas the REM AHI was not (P = .128).

Blood Pressure and Snoring

Snoring based on parent report is commonly used as a risk factor for SDB in children. In our study, snoring was identified based on two different methods.[3] The first method was a subjective assessment based on the survey in the Phase I study of snoring (moderate to severe) that was reported by the parent in 14.9% of the children. Subjective snoring was reported in 14.3% of those with an AHI < 1, 15.5% of those with an AHI between 1–5, and 37.5% of those with an AHI ≥ 5 (P = .181). The second measure of snoring was based on the objective evaluation obtained during the PSG and was present in 25.4% of the children. Objective snoring was observed in 20.9% of those with an AHI < 1, 36.6% of those with an AHI between1–5, and 75.0% of those with an AHI ≥ 5 (P <.001). We observed a general lack of agreement between these two estimates of snoring (κ =.109). The parental report of snoring versus no snoring was associated with borderline significantly higher systolic blood pressure 112.3 ± 1.1 versus 110.2 ± 0.4 mm Hg (P = .071), whereas the objectively measured snoring versus no snoring was associated with a significantly higher systolic blood pressure (112.2 ± 0.8 versus 109.9 ± 0.5 mm Hg, P = .017). The parent's report of snore versus no snore was not associated with an increased diastolic blood pressure (65.7 ± 0.8 versus 65.6 ± 0.3 mm Hg, P = .962) in contrast to the objective estimate (66.9 ± 0.5 versus 65.2

± 0.3 mm Hg, $P = .016$). Because of the stronger association of objective snoring with blood pressure, we examined whether objectively measured snoring modifies the AHI and elevated blood pressure association. Although the interaction between snoring and AHI was not significant, largely due to very small differences between snorers and non-snorers in the non-SDB (AHI < 1) group and very small sample size in the moderate SDB (AHI ≥ 5) group, we observed that snoring in the presence of mild-SDB may be associated with additional risk for elevated blood pressure, especially diastolic blood pressure.

Blood Pressure is Associated with Apnea/Hypopnea Indices

We assessed the mean levels of blood pressure across SDB categories (AHI < 1, AHI 1–5 and AHI ≥ 5) using ANCOVA.[3] In the final model adjusting for sampling weight, age, minority, sex, BMI percentile, sleep efficiency, snoring, and percentage of REM sleep, the mean systolic blood pressure levels (mean ± SE) by SDB categories were 109.9 ± 0.5, 111.7 ± 0.8, and 123.6 ± 3.7 mm Hg ($P = .001$ for trend), and for diastolic blood pressure were 65.6 ± 0.4, 65.5 ± 0.6, and 69.9 ± 2.8 mm Hg ($P = .136$ for trend), respectively.

In the final step of this analysis we evaluated the association of blood pressure and risk factors including: age, gender, minority, BMI percentiles (or waist circumference and height), REM percent, sleep efficiency, objective snoring, and AHI.[3] Older age, BMI percentile, waist circumference, height, and AHI were significantly associated with systolic blood pressure. However, only older age, BMI percentile, height, sleep efficiency, and snoring were significantly associated with diastolic blood pressure. It is worth noting that the effects of these risk factors on blood pressure were modeled mathematically adjusting for the effects of SDB, thus representing their respective effects on blood pressure independent of SDB status.

Our study suggests that SDB is an independent risk factor for elevated blood pressure in children aged 5 to 12 years.[3] At a threshold of AHI ≥ 5, the effect on blood pressure appears to warrant therapeutic intervention for SDB. Additional research is needed to assess the efficacy of SDB treatment on reducing blood pressure. At a threshold of AHI ≥ 3, the assessment of the blood pressure and the AHI in regular follow-up visits may be warranted. Again, future research is indicated to validate this suggestion. REM AHI does not appear to be a better predictor of blood pressure than the overall AHI. Primary snoring or snoring in the moderate group does not appear

to be a risk factor for blood pressure; however, snoring may be an additive factor for mild AHI. Finally, the association of waist circumference with systolic blood pressure supports the influence of metabolic factors in childhood SDB. AHI remained significantly associated with blood pressure after adjusting for these metabolic factors. This indicates that SDB in children is independently associated with elevated blood pressure, at least partially, via some nonobesity related pathways.

ASSOCIATION BETWEEN NEUROCOGNITIVE IMPAIRMENT AND SLEEP-DISORDERED BREATHING IN CHILDREN

Clinically, it is commonly assumed that neurocognitive impairment is a primary clinical outcome associated with childhood SDB. To assess this question, we evaluated all children who completed the neuropsychologic tests and had a full scale IQ greater than 80, resulting in a sample of 571.[21] Children diagnosed with medical problems, mental health disorders, or learning disabilities were not excluded from the study. In this sample, we identified six subjects (1%) as moderate SDB (AHI ≥ 5), 152 (26.6%) as mild SDB (1 ≤ AHI < 5), and 413 (72.3%) without SDB (AHI < 1). Significant differences across the three SDB groups were observed in terms of race, but not in terms of age, gender, or parent occupation (socioeconomic status). None of the children with moderate SDB were considered minority, while 31% of those with mild SDB and 20% in the group with no SDB were minority. The three AHI groups were assessed for differences on all neuropsychologic measures (intelligence, verbal and nonverbal reasoning ability, attention, executive functioning, memory, processing speed, and visual–motor skill). The one significant difference among the three groups was nonverbal IQ, however, the highest nonverbal IQ was observed in the moderate SDB group. All correlations between neuropsychologic test scores and continuous AHI were nonsignificant and the explained variance was small ($r^2 \leq .01$). Additional analyses were conducted to investigate the association between breathing-related arousals and neuropsychologic test scores, minimum degree of oxygen desaturation and test scores, as well as apnea index and test scores. All correlations between these additional variables and neuropsychologic test scores were nonsignificant and explained variance was small ($r^2 < .03$).

Although many previous studies have reported positive findings between children with moderate to severe SDB and neuropsychologic functioning,[22–26] our study suggests that children between the ages of 6–12 with mild SDB are not susceptible to neuropsychologic deficits. The strongest support for the position that SDB causes neurocognitive and behavioral deficits is found in a study[27] demonstrating improvement in cognitive test scores following adenotonsillectomy in children with mild to moderate SDB, and in three additional studies[5,26,28] demonstrating improvement in behavior and attention postsurgery. It is not possible, however, to conduct blind, placebo-controlled studies in such samples and therefore it is not known if the reported improvement in attention and cognition in these pre/post studies is the result of placebo effects or regression to the mean rather than as a result of treatment effects. The most parsimonious explanation for the differences between our study results and others is the lack of children with moderate SDB in our sample (n = 6) that limited our power. It is certainly reasonable to assume that the more severe the SDB, the more impact on neuropsychologic functioning.

The exact mechanisms by which SDB and reported neuropsychologic impairment may be associated remain unknown. Recently, however, several researchers have suggested that the mechanisms are most likely multifactorial.[2,29–31] For example, one study found that children with severe SDB and low IQs (≤85) had significantly higher levels of C-reactive protein (CRP, a serum marker of inflammation) than children with severe SDB and normal IQs.[29] This suggests that low IQ may be associated more strongly with systemic inflammation than SDB per se. Perhaps children present with different types of severe SDB: those with inflammation and associated neuropsychologic impairment (subtype 1) and those without inflammation and neuropsychologic impairment (subtype 2). Differences between subtypes in underlying medical conditions (eg, visceral adiposity, metabolic syndrome), or protective mechanisms (eg, genetics) may make some children more or less resilient to the effects of SDB and in turn neuropsychologic impairment. More robust associations between SDB and neuropsychologic functioning may result from the additive effect of genetic, metabolic, and environmental risk factors.

PREVALENCE OF RISK FACTORS FOR SLEEP-DISORDERED BREATHING IN CHILDREN

The sample of 700 children in our cohort consisted of 52.2% girls.[4] The age range was 5–12 years with an average age of 111.0 ± 0.8 months. Approximately one quarter (23.8%) of our sample was minority (Black not Hispanic = 13.8%, Hispanic = 6.3%). Our sample tended to be taller than expected with an average height percentile of 58.6 ± 1.1 as well as heavier with an average weight percentile of 61.1 ± 1.1. The average AHI was 0.8 ± 0.06 with a maximum value of 24.6 and an interquartile range of 0.85.

The analysis of the prevalence and risk factors for SDB categorized the subjects into four SDB categories (no SDB [AHI < 1 + no snore], primary snore [snore + AHI < 1], mild [1 ≤ AHI < 5], and moderate [AHI ≥ 5]), The prevalence of AHI ranged from 15.5% for primary snore, 25.0% for mild SDB, and 1.2% for moderate SDB. The distribution of the potential risk factors for SDB suggest that minority, BMI, waist circumference, tonsil size, nasal drainage, turbinate hypertrophy, and long soft palate were significantly associated with AHI. Factors that were clearly not associated with SDB included middle ear effusion, abnormal uvula, macroglossia, retrognathia, chronic cough and wheeze (all P >.30).

In order to establish the relative independent contribution of these risk factors we analyzed these data from a multivariate perspective using a stepwise logistic regression (retention criteria P <.05). We included in the initial models all variables with a univariate association of P <.30, which included gender, age, minority, BMI percentile, waist, tonsil size, mouth breathing, nasal drainage, turbinate hypertrophy, cervical adenopathy, long soft palate, abnormal palate, chronic sinusitis, and enuresis. We assessed the three levels of SDB each compared with no SDB. These systematic models enabled us to identify changing patterns of association at various thresholds of severity of SDB. In general, waist circumference appeared to be consistently retained as a significant predictor of SDB at all levels of severity. At the lowest threshold (ie, primary snoring) an association with waist circumference, age (negative), cervical adenopathy, and minority was observed. With mild SDB, waist, nasal abnormalities (eg, chronic sinusitis/rhinitis, turbinate hypertrophy, nasal drain), and minority were the significant risk factors. Finally, with moderate SDB, waist and long soft palate were identified as risk factors. At no level was tonsil size, as assessed by visual inspection, retained as a significant risk factor for SDB.

Previous estimates using this same threshold (AHI ≥ 5) have varied greatly ranging from 0.9% to 13.0%.[2,32,33] A major reason for this wide range of estimates may be due to small sample sizes of previous studies, varied criteria for SDB, and differences in the age range. We found only one study that used AHI ≥ 5 and a roughly similar age range (8–11 years), and it reported a prevalence of 0.9%.[2] This study was based on a cross-sectional sample which oversampled preterm and African American children. The final analysis of this study, however, only evaluated the independent contribution of race, preterm status, and BMI.

Because our analyses assessed a wide range of potential risk factors, possible etiologic mechanisms can be proposed. First, at milder AHI thresholds, nasal anatomic factors were more predominant (eg, chronic sinusitis/rhinitis, turbinate hypertrophy, nasal drain). As such, these factors were significant predictors of milder SDB in this population-based sample. In adults with SDB, it has been shown that systemic and local inflammatory mechanisms are an important contributing factor.[32] Treatment of nasal congestion in children with SDB with anti-inflammatory agents has been demonstrated to be effective with several compounds.[33–36] These data combined with the findings of this study suggest that a thorough evaluation and treatment of nasal abnormalities may be beneficial for this category of SDB in children.

Second, several studies have reported that obesity is a risk factor for SDB in children.[2,37,38] Obesity in children as in adults is associated with an increased risk for SDB. In addition, there are reports of increased adipose tissue in the uvula as well as in the soft palate.[39]

Third, in our study, waist circumference, but not neck circumference, was a consistent predictor of SDB at all levels of severity. This finding suggests that in children as in adults metabolic factors may play a contributing role in the mechanism of SDB. Moreover, it can be argued that the previous finding of BMI being independently associated with the failure of surgical treatment of SDB in children[40] further supports the hypothesis of a metabolic mechanism for SDB in children. Adipose tissue is capable of producing the proinflammatory molecule TNF[41] and systemic administration of TNF in animal models has been shown to be associated with a reduced muscle and diaphragm contractility.[42–45] In adult humans systemic administration of a TNF antagonist (etanercept) was associated with a reduction of both apnea and sleepiness.[46] Further support for the systemic inflammation mechanism associated with SDB in children comes from the finding that C-reactive protein[47,48] and plasma adherence molecules[49] have also been reported to be elevated in these children. In adults, it has been demonstrated that metabolic factors are associated with SDB, which may be the mechanism for the cardiovascular risk observed in these patients. Similarly, in children with SDB it has been reported that fasting insulin levels independent of BMI are associated with the severity of SDB.[50,51]

SUMMARY

From a clinical standpoint, professionals who evaluate and treat children with SDB should be cognizant of comorbid risk factors associated with this disorder. Based on a representative sample we have observed that cardiovascular risk is a primary risk factor for SDB in children as in adults. Specifically, in the Penn State Child Cohort an AHI $\geq$ 5 but not an AI $\geq$ 1 was associated with significantly elevated blood pressure whereas an AHI $\geq$ 3 was associated with a borderline significant increase in blood pressure. Our study suggests that children ages 5–12 with mild SDB are likely not to be at risk for neuropsychologic impairment and the coexistence of mild SDB with any neuropsychologic impairment should be considered comorbid and not necessarily causal. Certainly, there may be individual children for whom mild SDB affects neuropsychologic functioning, but for a large group of community children, mild SDB was not significantly related to neuropsychologic functioning. The AHI calculated within REM does not appear to be a strong risk factor for elevated blood pressure. In terms of snoring the parent report does not appear to be a strong predictor of risk for elevated blood pressure, whereas snoring observed objectively during the PSG is a better predictor. Based on the association with increased blood pressure the threshold of AHI $\geq$ 5 appears to warrant therapeutic treatment for SDB in children. At a threshold of AHI $\geq$ 3 the assessment of blood pressure and regular follow-up visits may be warranted. We observed a prevalence of 1.2% for moderate SDB based on a threshold of AHI $\geq$ 5 in elementary school children (K–5). Waist circumference and BMI were the consistent independent risk factors across several thresholds of severity of SDB. This suggests that, in children as in adults, metabolic and inflammatory factors may be an important mechanism in the development of SDB, implying that adenotonsillectomy may not always be the best first line treatment. Finally, nasal abnormalities (eg, chronic sinusitis/rhinitis) were significant risk factors in children with milder SDB, suggesting that the evaluation and treatment of these abnormalities might be beneficial for this category of patients. Future research is indicated to confirm these findings, especially in children with moderate to severe SDB. Ultimately, we believe that the mechanism for SDB in children are complex and likely share many of the etiologic risk factors with adults.

REFERENCES

1. Enright PL, Goodwin JL, Sherril DL, et al. Blood-pressure elevation associated with sleep-related breathing disorder in a community sample of White and Hispanic. Arch Pediatr Adolesc Med 2003; 157:901–4.

2. Rosen CL, Larkin EK, Kirchner L, et al. Prevalence and risk factors for sleep-disordered breathing in 8- to 11-year-old children: association with race and prematurity. J Pediatr 2003;142:383–9.

3. Bixler EO, Vgontzas AN, Lin H-M, et al. Blood pressure associated with sleep-disordered breathing in a population sample of children. Hypertension 2008;52:841–6.

4. Bixler EO, Vgontzas AN, Lin H-M, et al. Sleep-disordered breathing in children in a general population sample: prevalence and risk factors. Sleep 2009, in press.

5. Ali NJ, Pitson DJ, Stradling JR. Snoring, sleep disturbance, and behaviour in 4–5 year olds. Arch Dis Child 1993;68:360–6.

6. Rechtschaffen A, Kales A. A manual of standardized terminology, techniques and scoring system for sleep stages of human subjects. NIMH Publication 204. Washington, DC: U.S. Government Printing Office; 1968.

7. Wechsler D. Wechsler abbreviated scale of intelligence. The Psychological Corporation: San Antonio (TX) 1999.

8. Mariani MA, Barkley RA. Neuropsychological and academic functioning in preschool boys with attention deficit hyperactivity disorder. Dev Neuropsychol 1997;13:111–29.

9. Brocki KC, Bohlin G. Executive functions in children aged 6 to 13: a dimensional and developmental study. Dev Neuropsychol 2004;26:571–93.

10. Mayes SD, Calhoun SL. The Gordon diagnostic system and WISC-III freedom from distractibility index: validity in identifying clinic-referred children with and without ADHD. Psychol Rep 2002;91:575–87.

11. Mayes SD, Calhoun SL. WISC-IV and WISC-III profiles in children with ADHD. J Atten Disord 2006;9:486–93.

12. Mayes SD, Calhoun SL. Analysis of WISC-III, Stanford-Binet IV, and academic achievement test scores in children with autism. J Autism Dev Disord 2003;33:329–41.

13. Calhoun SL, Mayes SD. Processing speed in children with clinical disorders. Psychol Sch 2005;42:333–43.

14. Koren R, Kofman O, Berger A. Analysis of word clustering in verbal fluency of school-aged children. Arch Clin Neuropsychol 2005;20:1087–104.

15. Donders J. Structural equation analysis of the California verbal learning test – children's version in the standardization sample. Dev Neuropsychol 1999;15:395–406.

16. Mottram L, Donders J. Cluster subtypes on the California verbal learning test-children's version after pediatric traumatic brain injury. Dev Neuropsychol 2006;30:865–83.

17. Golden CJ, Freshwater SM, Golden GL. Stroop color and word test – children's version. Wood Dale (IL): Stoelting; 2003.

18. Jensen AR, Rohwer WD Jr. The Stroop color word test: a review. Acta Psychol (Amst) 1966;25:36–93.

19. Chase-Carmichael CA, Ris MD, Weber AM, et al. Neurologic validity of the Wisconsin card sorting test with a pediatric population. Clin Neuropsychol 1999;13:405–13.

20. Goh DY, Galster P, Marcus CL. Sleep architecture and respiratory disturbances in children with obstructive sleep apnea. Am J Respir Crit Care Med 2000;162:682–6.

21. Calhoun SL, Mayes SD, Vgontzas AN, et al. No relationship between neurocognitive functioning and mild sleep-disordered breathing in a community sample of children. J Clin Sleep Med (in press).

22. O'Brien L, Mervis CB, Holbrook CR, et al. Neurobehavioral implications of habitual snoring in children. Pediatrics 2004;114(1):44–9.

23. Beebe DW, Wells C, Jeffries J, et al. Neuropsychological effects of pediatric obstructive sleep apnea. J Int Neuropsychol Soc 2004;10:962–75.

24. Halbower AC, Deganokar M, Barker PB, et al. Childhood obstructive sleep apnea associates with neuropsychological deficits and neuronal brain injury. PLoS Med 2006;3(8):1391–402.

25. Lewin DS, Rosen RC, England SJ, et al. Preliminary evidence of behavioral and cognitive sequelae of obstructive sleep apnea in children. Sleep Med 2002;3:5–13.

26. Anastopoulos AD, Spisto MA, Maher MC. The WISC-III Freedom from distractibility factor: its utility in identifying children with attention deficit hyperactivity disorder. Psychol Assess 1994;6: 368–71.

27. Friedman B-C, Hendeles-Amitai BA, Kozimnsky E, et al. Adenotonsillectomy improves neurocognitive function in children with obstructive sleep apnea syndrome. Sleep 2003;26(8):999–1005.

28. Chervin RD, Ruzicka DL, Giordani BJ, et al. Sleep disordered breathing, behavior, and cognition in children before and after adenotonsillectomy. Pediatrics 2006;117:e769–78.

29. Gozal D, Crabtree VM, Sans Capdevila O, et al. C-reactive protein, obstructive sleep apnea, and cognitive dysfunction in school-aged children. Am J Respir Crit Care Med 2007;176:188–93.

30. Kelly A, Marcus C. Childhood obesity, inflammation and apnea. Am J Respir Crit Care Med 2005;171: 202–3.

31. Spilsbury JC, Storfer-Isser A, Kirchner HL, et al. Neighborhood disadvantage as a risk factor for

pediatric obstructive sleep apnea. J Pediatr 2006; 149:342–7.

32. Vgontzas AN, Bixler EO, Chrousos GP. Sleep apnea is a manifestation of the metabolic syndrome. Sleep Med Rev 2005;9:211–24.

33. Brouillette RT, Manoukian JJ, Ducharme FM, et al. Efficacy of fluticasone nasal spray for pediatric obstructive sleep apnea. J Pediatr 2001;138:838–44.

34. Mansfield LE, Gonzolo D, Posey CR, et al. Sleep disordered breathing and daytime quality of life in children with allergic rhinitis during treatment with intranasal budesonide. Ann Allergy Asthma Immunol 2004;92:240–4.

35. Goldbart AD, Goldman JL, Veiling MC, et al. Leukotriene modifier therapy for mild sleep-disordered breathing in children. Am J Respir Crit Care Med 2005;172:364–70.

36. Kheirandish L, Goldbart AD, Gozal D. Intranasal steroids and oral leukotriene modifier therapy in residual sleep-disordered breathing after tonsillectomy and adenoidectomy in children. Pediatrics 2006;117:61–6.

37. O'Brien LM, Sitha S, Baur LA, et al. Obesity increases the risk of persisting obstructive sleep apnea after treatment in children. Int J Pediatr Otorhinolaryngol 2006;70:1555–60.

38. Redline S, Tishler OV, Schlucter M, et al. Risk factors for sleep-disordered breathing in children: associations with obesity, race and respiratory problems. Am J Respir Crit Care Med 1999;159:1527–32.

39. Stauffer JL, Buick MK, Bixler EO, et al. Morphology of the uvula in obstructive sleep apnea. Am Rev Respir Dis 1989;107:724–8.

40. Tauman R, Gulliver TE, Krishna J, et al. Persistence of obstructive sleep apnea syndrome in children after adenotonsillectomy. J Pediatr 2006;149:803–8.

41. Hotamisligil GS, Shargill NS, Spiegelman BM. Adipose expression of tumor necrosis factor-α:

direct role in obesity-linked insulin resistance. Science 1993;259:87–91.

42. Wilcox PG, Wakai Y, Walley KR, et al. Tumor necrosis factor alpha decreases in vivo diaphragm contractility in dogs. Am J Respir Crit Care Med 1994;150:1368–73.

43. Wilcox P, Milliken C, Bressler B. High-dose tumor necrosis factor alpha produces an impairment of hamster diaphragm contractility. Am J Respir Crit Care Med 1996;153:1611–5.

44. Li X, Moody MR, Engel D, et al. Cardiac-specific overexposure of tumor necrosis factor α causes oxidative stress and contractile dysfunction in mouse diaphragm. Circulation 2000;102:1690–6.

45. Reid MB, Laannergren J, Westerblad H. Respiratory and limb muscle weakness induced by tumor necrosis factor α. Am J Respir Crit Care Med 2002;166:479–84.

46. Vgontzas AN, Zoumakis E, Lin HM, et al. Marked decrease in sleepiness in patients with sleep apnea by etanercept, a tumor necrosis factor-alpha antagonist. J Clin Endocrinol Metab 2004;89(9):4409–13.

47. Larkin EK, Rosen CL, Kirchner L, et al. Variation of C-reactive protein levels in adolescents association with sleep-disordered breathing and sleep duration. Circulation 2005;111:1978–84.

48. Taumen R, Ivanenko A, O'Brien LM, et al. Plasma C-reactive protein levels among children with sleep-disordered breathing. Pediatrics 2004;113: e564–9.

49. O'Brien LM, Serpero LD, Tauman R, et al. Plasma adhesion molecules in children with sleep-disordered breathing. Chest 2006;129:947–53.

50. de la Eva RC, Baur LA, Donaghue KC, et al. Metabolic correlates with obstructive sleep apnea in obese subjects. J Pediatr 2002;140:654–9.

51. Li AM, Chan MH, Chan DF, et al. Insulin and obstructive sleep apnea in obese children. Pediatr Pulmonol 2006;41:1175–81.

Outcomes from the Tucson Children's Assessment of Sleep Apnea Study

Rohit Budhiraja, MD[a], Stuart F. Quan, MD[b,c],*

KEYWORDS

- Sleep-disordered breathing • Children • Epidemiology
- Learning • Hypertension • Behavior
- Ventilatory drive • TuCASA

That sleep-disordered breathing (SDB) occurs in children has long been known. However, emerging recognition of the frequent occurrence and impact of SDB in the pediatric population has led to an increased clinical and academic interest in this condition. The presenting symptoms of childhood SDB include snoring, arousals, enuresis, restlessness during sleep, daytime sleepiness, and hyperactivity.[1,2] Of particular importance is that, unlike SDB in adults, hyperactivity and not daytime sleepiness may be the most evident manifestation. Moreover, the presence of SDB has been suggested to result in an adverse impact on neurobehavioral development.[3–6]

The Tucson Children's Assessment of Sleep Apnea (TuCASA) study is a prospective cohort study aimed at assessing the objective prevalence of SDB in preadolescent children aged 6 to 12 years using polysomnography (PSG). Although some studies have evaluated the presence of symptoms and correlates of SDB in Caucasian and African American children,[7] TuCASA is the first one to study a large population of Hispanic children. Further, the study has investigated the symptoms, anatomic or physiologic correlates,

and consequences of SDB, including neuropsychologic performance, in children. This article examines the methodologic procedures and the cross-sectional outcome data from this study.

STUDY DESIGN
Participants

The study design for TuCASA has been described in detail previously.[8] Five hundred three 6- to 12-year-old Caucasian and Hispanic children were recruited from selected elementary schools in the Tucson Unified School District to undergo unattended home PSG. Incentives were offered to schools to encourage participation. The selected schools were prescreened to ensure that between 25% and 75% of their children were of Hispanic descent. The children were asked to take home a short screening questionnaire with sleep, anthropometric, and demographic items. Parents were requested to complete the questionnaire, return it to the investigators, and indicate whether they would allow study personnel to call them. The screening questionnaire consisted of a one-page survey designed to assess the severity of

The Tucson Children's Assessment of Sleep Apnea Study is supported by the National Heart, Lung, and Blood Institute grant HL 62373.

[a] Section of Pulmonary and Critical Care Medicine, Southern Arizona VA Healthcare System and University of Arizona College of Medicine, 3601 South 6th Avenue, Tucson, AZ 85723, USA

[b] Department of Medicine, Arizona Respiratory Center, University of Arizona College of Medicine, 1501 N. Campbell Avenue, Tucson, AZ 85724, USA

[c] Division of Sleep Medicine, Brigham and Women's Hospital, Harvard Medical School, 401 Park Drive, 2nd Floor East, Boston, MA 02215, USA

* Corresponding author. Division of Sleep Medicine, Harvard Medical School, 401 Park Drive, 2nd Floor East, Boston, MA 02215.

E-mail address: squan@arc.arizona.edu (S.F. Quan).

Sleep Med Clin 4 (2009) 9–18
doi:10.1016/j.jsmc.2008.11.002
1556-407X/08/$ – see front matter © 2009 Elsevier Inc. All rights reserved.

obstructive sleep apnea syndrome (OSAS)-related symptoms in children. Questions such as "How often does your child snore loudly?," "Is your child sleepy during the daytime?," "Does your child stop breathing during sleep?," and "Does your child have learning problems?" were evaluated by a parent on the scale of never, rarely, occasionally, frequently, almost always, or don't know. A total of 7055 questionnaires were distributed, with a 33% return rate. Of the children for whom the surveys were returned, 45.4% were Hispanic and 38% were Caucasian. Of those returning questionnaires, 1219 (52.4%) supplied recruitment information, and from this group, 503 children were selected to undergo unattended home PSG. Children who had chronic medical conditions and attention deficit hyperactivity disorder (ADHD) were excluded. A full unattended PSG was performed at the home within 1 month of recruitment and another visit was scheduled at the medical center for neurocognitive evaluation several weeks later.

Home Polysomnography

A two-person, mixed-gender team arrived at the participant's home approximately 1 hour before the child's regular bedtime to prepare the child for an unattended PSG using a portable monitor capable of recording a full PSG montage.[9] Use of this system in TuCASA has been described in detail elsewhere.[8] Briefly, sensors included C3/A2 and C4/A1 electroencephalogram, right and left electro-oculogram, a bipolar submental electromyogram, thoracic and abdominal displacement (inductive plethysmography bands), airflow (nasal/oral thermistor), nasal pressure cannula, oximetry, ECG (single bipolar lead), snoring (microphone attached to the vest), body position (Hg gauge sensor), and ambient light (sensor attached to the vest to record on/off). The thermistor and nasal pressure signals were collected simultaneously by taping a nasal/oral thermistor on the superior surface of a nasal cannula. The data from the PSG were stored in real time on a 40-MB Personal Computer Memory Card International Association (PCMCIA) flashcard and reviewed in the morning. If the study had insufficient duration or quality of artifact-free signal, fewer than 4 hours of oximetry, or equipment malfunction, it was categorized as a failed study. A study was classified as "good" if a minimum of 5 or more hours of signal were scorable on at least two respiratory channels (airflow, thoracic or abdominal bands), oximetry, and one electroencephalogram signal. If 4 to 5 hours of scorable signal were present on at least one electroencephalogram, oximeter, and respiratory signal, the study was

classified as "fair." If an initial study failed, the subject was asked to have another sleep recording. The final overall "pass rate" of the studies was 97%.

Sleep was manually staged according to Rechtschaffen and Kales criteria.[10] Arousals were identified using criteria published by the American Academy of Sleep Medicine.[11] Obstructive apneas were identified if the magnitude of any ventilation signal decreased to below 25% of the baseline amplitude for at least 6 seconds or for two or more consecutive breaths. Hypopneas were scored if the magnitude of any ventilation signal decreased to below approximately 70% of the baseline amplitude for at least 6 seconds or for two or more consecutive breaths. Central apneas were scored if airflow and thoracoabdominal effort were absent. To describe a respiratory disturbance index (RDI) defined by different magnitudes of oxygen desaturation or arousal, software linked various levels of minimum oxygen desaturation or the presence of arousal to each scored apneic or hypopneic event. In this way, an RDI could be generated characterized by no oxygen desaturation (RDI0) or by 2% (RDI2%), 3% (RDI3%), or an arousal (RDI-A).

To assess the reliability of scoring, 5% of studies were rescored by the same scorer on a blinded basis. No significant difference was found between initial and repeat scoring. The two sets of studies showed good agreement regarding classification as sleep apnea (RDI0<1 or $\geq$1, κ = 0.78). A night-to-night variability study in 10 children showed no statistically significant differences in key sleep parameters between two different nights of recording.

During the home visit, a visual oropharynx inspection was done, anthropometric measurements, seated blood pressure (BP), and a digital photograph of the oropharynx and tonsils were taken, and a more extensive sleep habits questionnaire was completed, in addition to PSG. A poststudy survey was completed by the caregiver the morning after the PSG.

Behavioral Evaluation

Behavior problems were measured using the Conners' Parent Rating Scale–Revised (CPRS-R) long version (L) and the Child Behavior Checklist (CBCL). Families were paid $25 for completing the behavioral evaluation. The long version of CPRS-R contains 80 items.[12] It is typically used with parents or caregivers when comprehensive information and *Diagnostic and Statistical Manual of Mental Disorders* (Fourth Edition) (*DSM-IV*) consideration are required. Scales include oppositional, cognitive problems, inattention, hyperactivity, anxious-shy, perfectionism, social problems, psychosomatic, Conners' Global Index (restless impulsive, emotional lability), *DSM-IV* symptom subscales (inattentive, hyperactive impulsive), and ADHD index. Parents rate their children's behavior in the past month on a four-point Likert scale (not true at all; just a little true; pretty much true; very much true). Subscale T scores can be calculated based on a large age- and gender-specific normative sample. A T score (mean 50, standard deviation [SD] 10) higher than 65 is considered to indicate moderate-to-severe clinical impairment. The CBCL was designed to assess social competence and behavior problems in children aged 4 to 18.[13] It includes 118 items related to behavior problems, which are scored on a three-point scale (not true, somewhat true, or very/often true).

Neurocognitive Evaluation

A neurocognitive assessment was performed a mean of 38 days after the successful completion of the PSG. The 3-hour assessment battery consisted of a series of standardized neurocognitive measures completed in a fixed order and ending with a single standard 10-minute visual psychomotor vigilance task (PVT) trial.[14,15] The cognitive measures administered to the children were completed as follows: the Wechsler Abbreviated Scale of Intelligence (WASI);[16] letter–word identification, applied problems, and dictation from the Woodcock-Johnson Psycho-Educational Battery–Revised Tests of Achievement (WJ–R);[17] and the Children's Auditory Verbal Learning Test-2.[18] Dependent measures from each of these tests are age-based standard scores that have a mean of 100 and SD of 15, and higher scores indicate better performance. The WASI is a brief and reliable measure of

intelligence and was used to facilitate characterization of the study participants. Measures of full-scale intelligence quotient (IQ), verbal IQ, and performance IQ were obtained. The WJ–R was used to measure academic achievement measures were used to assess learning of, and memory for, information learned before and outside of the evaluation setting. Letter–word identification assesses letter and single word reading. Applied problems assesses math skills. Dictation is a measure of spelling, punctuation, grammar, and word usage. The Children's Auditory Verbal Learning Test-2[18] was used to measure auditory verbal learning and memory abilities. This multi-trial word list learning task provides age-based standard scores for each of the following: five list learning trials, overall learning across trials (level of learning), recall of a second word list (interference trial) presented after the learning trials, and immediate and delayed recall of the original list. Attention was evaluated using the CPRS-R (L) questionnaire. The PVT-192 was used for the psychomotor vigilance testing. It is a simple task administered on a handheld device. Participants were asked to press a button as quickly as possible each time they saw a visual stimulus appear (a small red light-emitting diode–digital counter). The stimulus was presented approximately 100 times during the 10-minute task, with the interstimulus interval varying randomly from 2 to 10 seconds.

BASELINE CHARACTERISTICS OF THE TUCSON CHILDREN'S ASSESSMENT OF SLEEP APNEA COHORT

Five hundred three children underwent PSG in the TuCASA study. The baseline characteristics of this sample are shown in **Table 1**. Forty-nine percent of the children were Hispanic and half the subjects were girls. The mean body mass index (BMI) was

Table 1
Baseline characteristics of the Tucson Children's Assessment of Sleep Apnea cohort

	Age (y)			
	All	**≤7**	**8–9**	**≥10**
Total cohort	503	165	184	154
Boys/girls (%)	50/50	53/47	49/51	49/51
Caucasians/Hispanic (%)	59/41	59/41	59/41	56/44
BMI (mean ± SD)	18 ± 9	17 ± 4	18 ± 3	19 ± 5
Obese (%)	10.4	11.4	8.3	9.2
Neck circumference, cm (mean ± SD)	27 ± 3	26 ± 3	27 ± 4	29 ± 3

Abbreviations: BMI, body mass index; SD, standard deviation.

18.0 kg/m^2 (SD 4.4) and 10.4% had a BMI greater than the 95th percentile for their age, sex, and ethnicity and were classified as "obese." Of the 503 PSGs, 480 were found to be of good quality and were used for further analyses. The average total time in bed was 542.7 ± 85.7 minutes, sleep latency was 18.5 ± 21.0 minutes, and total sleep time was 487.0 ± 79.7 minutes, with the average sleep efficiency being 89.8%.[8] These values were not significantly different in boys and girls.

SLEEP-DISORDERED BREATHING
Prevalence and Predictors of Sleep-Disordered Breathing

The primary goal of the TuCASA study was to determine the prevalence and correlates of SDB. The children were diagnosed as having SDB if the RDI3% was greater than or equal to one per hour of total sleep time. Composite variables were created based on a combination of selected survey items from the basic screening questionnaire and the more extensive sleep-habits questionnaire to elucidate the clinical correlates of SDB.[19]

The children were classified as snorers if parents reported that their child snored loudly "frequently" or "almost always." Witnessed apnea was defined by the parents' positive reply to the following items on the questionnaire: their child stopped or struggled to breathe, their child's lips turned blue, or they shook their child because they were worried about their child's breathing during sleep "frequently" or "almost always." Subjects were diagnosed as having excessive daytime sleepiness (EDS) if the parents answered "frequently" or "almost always" on any of the following: their child was sleepy in the daytime, fell asleep while watching TV or in school, or had problems with falling asleep during the day. Insomnia was diagnosed if the parents reported that their child had trouble falling or staying asleep, did not have enough sleep, or was troubled by waking up too early and not being able to get back to sleep. Learning problems were considered present if the parent reported that the child had a problem with learning frequently or almost always.

Of the children undergoing PSG, 15% had snoring, 5.2% had witnessed apnea, 16.3% had EDS, 29.4% had insomnia, and 5.8% had learning problems.[8] PSG evidence of SDB (RDI3% ≥ 1) was present in 24% of children (mean RDI3% 2.6 ± 3.4). The mean RDI3% in children who did not have SDB was 0.38 ± 0.28. The likelihood of SDB was higher in boys than in girls (odds ratio [OR] 1.9, CI 1.2–3.0, P = .006). Snoring (OR 3.5, CI 2.0–6.2, P = .001) and EDS (OR 2.1, CI 1.2–3.8, P = .01) were also

significantly associated with SDB. Furthermore, learning problems, as reported by parents, were more common in children who had SDB than in those who did not have SDB (11.3% versus 4.1%, P = .004). However, reported witnessed apneas (OR 1.8, CI 0.8–4.3, P = .15) or insomnia (OR 0.9, CI 0.6–1.5, P = .85) were not associated with a higher likelihood of SDB. In addition, ethnicity (Hispanic or Caucasian), age, obesity, and airway size were not significantly different between children who did or did not have SDB.

Analyses were performed to assess the sensitivity, specificity, and likelihood ratios of different predictors for SDB.[8] The sensitivity of different variables for identifying SDB was usually low, with highest being that of male sex (60%). Frequent loud snoring, EDS, and learning problems had low sensitivities of 29.5%, 24.4%, and 11.3%, respectively. The sensitivities continued to be low when combinations of different symptoms or demographic variables were assessed. However, the specificities of learning problems (95.9%), snoring (89.5%), and EDS (86.3%) for SDB were high. Similarly, the combinations of snoring and learning problems (98.9%), snoring and EDS (97.0%), and snoring and male gender (95.1%) had high specificities for SDB.

These findings should be useful in the clinical evaluation of children who have possible SDB. They suggest that although many children who have SDB will not have habitual snoring and EDS, when the symptoms are present, a diagnosis of SDB should be sought. Positive likelihood ratios for snoring (2.8) and learning problems (2.8) again suggest an increase in the chance of SDB being present when these are present. The results of the study also add to the current literature suggesting SDB as a possible contributing factor to poor academic achievement in children.

One limitation of the TuCASA study is the use of only a thermistor to monitor airflow. Because an end-tidal carbon dioxide (CO_2) monitor was not used, it is possible that some cases of obstructive hypoventilation may have been missed. Moreover, use of a nasal pressure transducer to identify hypopneas during PSG is now considered standard practice.[20] Because most TuCASA analyses used thermistor-derived recordings, the presence and severity of SDB may be underestimated. Indeed, a comparison of nasal pressure transducer and thermistor in a sample from the TuCASA cohort suggested that the former was able to detect a significantly higher number of events than the latter.[21] However, the nasal pressure transducer showed a greater likelihood of signal loss than the thermistor, which may make use of the former unfeasible in young children.

Sleep-Disordered Breathing and Learning

Kaemingk and colleagues[14] assessed the relationship between intelligence, learning, and memory, and academic achievement and SDB in TuCASA subjects. A group of children who had an RDI0 of greater than or equal to five (n = 77) was compared with a group who had an RDI0 of less than five (n = 72). A significant inverse relationship was evident between RDI0 and full IQ, performance IQ, immediate recall, and applied problems. Learning and memory were decreased in the group of otherwise healthy children who had a RDI0 of five or more. These results suggest that SDB has an important adverse impact on the ability to learn during childhood. Whether such impairment has lasting consequences will not be known until long-term follow-up of these children is completed.

Sleep-Disordered Breathing and Hypertension

Strong evidence implicates SDB as a risk factor for hypertension in adults.[22,23] However, the data assessing such an association in children have been meager. In TuCASA, BP measurements were performed on children during the home visit for PSG recording. BP was measured in triplicate from the right arm of the child using a portable mercury sphygmomanometer and standardized techniques.[24] The appropriate BP cuff was selected according to the measured arm circumference. In an analysis of the first 239 TuCASA study participants who completed unattended home PSGs, the association between hypertension and SDB was examined.[25] Boys constituted 55% of this sample and 51% of the children were Hispanic. The mean age was 8.7 years, the BMI was 18.2 kg/m^2, and the mean neck size was 27 cm. Obesity was defined as a BMI of greater than the 95th percentile standardized for age, sex, and ethnicity[26] and 12% of the children were obese by this criterion.

The mean $\pm$ SD systolic and diastolic BPs were 98.4 $\pm$ 10.6 mm Hg and 62.0 $\pm$ 8.9 mm Hg, respectively. BP elevation was systolic and diastolic BP was above the 90th percentile when adjusted for age, height, and sex.[27] Fifteen children (6%) had hypertension. Associations were noted between systolic and diastolic BP elevation and RDI defined by either 2%, 3%, or 4% oxygen desaturations linked with apneic and hypopneic events. However, BP elevation was not noted in children who had apneic/hypopneic events unassociated with oxygen desaturation. Obesity, poorer sleep efficiency, arousal index, and RDI2% were independently associated with diastolic BP elevation. Habitual loud snoring, witnessed apnea, RDI2%, and poorer sleep efficiency were associated with systolic BP elevation. Sex, ethnicity, total sleep time, and parental smoking were not associated with either systolic or diastolic hypertension.

This study provides evidence for the association between poor sleep and SDB and hypertension in children. The results were in accordance with a prior study that reported higher BP in children who had OSA compared with those with primary snoring.[28] That BP was not elevated in the absence of oxygen desaturation suggests hypoxemia to be a major factor in the cause of SDB-related hypertension. This finding is consistent with data in adults suggesting that hypoxemic stress may be the pivotal factor contributing to endothelial dysfunction, hypertension, and SDB.[29] Furthermore, obesity was associated with hypertension, suggesting that controlling obesity may help limit such adverse consequences.

Sleep-Disordered Breathing and Behavioral Problems

The correlation between SDB and behavioral problems was analyzed in one TuCASA study.[30] The mean RDI0 for the sample evaluated in this study was 5.29 (SD 4.80, range 0.10–72.4). Children in the upper 15% of the RDI distribution had higher mean CBCL scores on the aggressive, attention problems, social problems, thought problems, total and externalizing scales. Hyperactivity, however, was not strongly associated with a higher RDI. Similarly, on the CPRS-R, high ORs for oppositional, cognitive problems, social problems, psychosomatic problems, ADHD index, and *DSM* total scales were seen in children in the upper 15% of the RDI distribution. Other data from TuCASA indicate that snoring children also have a higher prevalence of behavioral problems (**Fig. 1**). These results indicate that SDB is associated with increased behavioral morbidity in children who have SDB. Furthermore, they are consistent with clinical observations that behavioral problems are frequently the primary or initial manifestation of SDB in children.

Parasomnias and Sleep-Disordered Breathing

Parasomnias in children have been associated with sleep disruption, SDB, psychiatric comorbidities, and distress to the child and the family members.[31–33] One TuCASA analysis characterized the relationship between parasomnias and SDB in these children. A sleep habits questionnaire administered on the night of PSG in this study included questions such as "Does this child sleepwalk?" and "Does this child talk in his or her

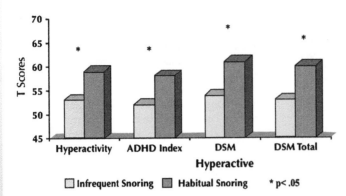

Fig. 1. T Scores on the Conners' Parent Rating Scales. Values are higher in snoring children.

sleep? (Talk without being fully awake?)" and "How often does this child awaken at night afraid or appearing tearful?" The choices of responses were "never," "less than three times per month," "three to five times per month," or "more than five times per month." A child was classified as having parasomnias if sleepwalking was present more than three times per month, sleep talking was present more than five times per month or if the child had more than five fearful awakenings per month. Enuresis was defined as occurring more than five times per month.[34]

Of the children undergoing PSG, 3.5% had sleepwalking, 11.3% had sleep talking, 6.3% had fearful awakenings, and 7.5% had enuresis.[8] Children with sleep talking were more likely to have concomitant sleepwalking and sleep terrors. However, arousal parasomnias and enuresis showed no association. Children with sleepwalking showed an increased prevalence of reported EDS, insomnia, and learning problems and a trend toward more habitual snoring.[34] Children with sleep talking were more likely to have habitual snoring, insomnia, and learning problems, but not EDS. Children with fearful awakenings were more likely to have habitual snoring, EDS, insomnia, and learning problems. Enuresis was strongly associated with habitual snoring and witnessed apnea. As shown in **Fig. 2**, sleepwalking (OR 2.9, CI 1.1–7.8, $P = .02$) and sleep talking (OR 2.2, CI 1.2–4.1, $P = .006$) were associated with a higher likelihood of SDB. The data showed a nonsignificant trend for enuresis to be associated with SDB (OR 1.9, CI 0.9–3.9, $P = .08$). Fearful awakenings or child being fidgety were not associated with SDB.[8]

Parasomnias such as sleepwalking and sleep talking have traditionally been considered usual and inconsequential childhood occurrences. However, the TuCASA study demonstrated a greater likelihood of SDB and other sleep symptoms and learning problems among children who had parasomnias. Parasomnias may be a result of SDB and can improve with treatment of SDB.[35] It remains to be elucidated whether the learning problems encountered in children who have parasomnias are a function of concomitant SDB or whether parasomnias are an independent risk factor for the learning difficulties.

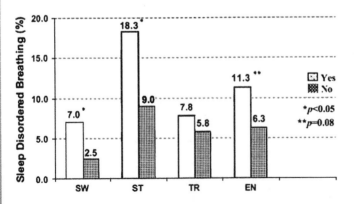

Fig. 2. Associations between sleep-disordered breathing (SDB) and parasomnias. SDB was defined as an RDI3% of more than one per hour of total sleep time. EN, enuresis; ST, sleep talking; SW, sleepwalking; TR, sleep terrors. (*From* Goodwin JL, Kaemingk KL, Fregosi RF, et al. Parasomnias and sleep disordered breathing in Caucasian and Hispanic children - the Tucson Children's Assessment of Sleep Apnea study. BMC Med 2004;2:14; with permission. Available at: http://www.biomedcentral.com/1741-7015/2/14. Accessed June 23, 2008. Published online 2004 April 28. doi: 10.1186/

Sleep-Disordered Breathing and Ventilatory Drive

Hypoxic and hypercapnic ventilatory drive in relation to the severity of SDB was examined in 50 children recruited from the TuCASA cohort.[36] The investigators assessed ventilatory drive by measuring the mouth occlusion pressure response (pressure at 0.1 second [$P_{0.1}$]) in normoxia, at two levels of isocapnic hypoxia, and at three levels of hyperoxic hypercapnia. They found a significant correlation between resting pressure of end-tidal CO_2 ($P_{ET}CO_2$) with the obstructive apnea-hypopnea index (OAHI). The hypoxic, but not the hypercapnic, occlusion pressure response was significantly related to the OAHI (**Fig. 3**). These results suggest that CO_2 retention and reduced hypoxic ventilatory drive occur in children who have a high OAHI. CO_2 retention during wakefulness in children who have severe SDB may be consequent to perturbed central ventilatory control. Although mechanical obstruction from enlarged tonsils causing a narrowing of the pharyngeal airway may contribute to CO_2 retention, a study demonstrating failure of adenotonsillectomy to abolish resting CO_2 retention during wakefulness in children who had SDB argues against this being a primary mechanism.[37] The reduced hypoxic responsiveness seen in children in the study may be a paraphenomenon of SDB or may predispose children to SDB.

Upper Airway Collapsibility in Sleep-Disordered Breathing

Children who have severe obstructive sleep apnea have a more collapsible pharynx than those of normal children.[38] Seventeen children from the TuCASA cohort underwent testing to assess whether children who have mild SDB composed primarily of hypopneas rather than apneas also have more collapsible airways than normal children.[39] Airway collapsibility was estimated in 7 children who had mild SDB (11.5 ± 0.1 hypopneas/h) and 10 age-matched controls (1.9 ± 0.2 hypopneas/h) during stable, non–rapid eye movement sleep. The groups were similar in regards to BMI, neck circumference, and estimated airway size. The intermittent Pcrit method (brief [two-breath] duration and sudden reductions in pharyngeal pressure by connecting the breathing mask to a negative pressure source) revealed more collapsible airways in children in the SDB group than in the age-matched controls. These observations point to an intrinsic abnormality in the pharyngeal airway of children who have even mild SDB that may predispose to this disorder.

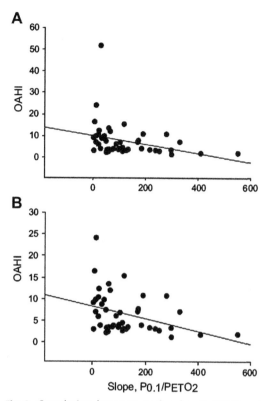

Fig. 3. Correlation between each subject's OAHI and the slope of the $P_{0.1}/P_{ET}O_2$ curve. The top panel (*A*) represents data from all subjects, and the bottom panel (*B*) shows that the relation is strengthened when the outlier with the very high OAHI is removed from the data set. The slope of the $P_{0.1}/P_{ET}O_2$ curves were obtained for each subject during the response tests $P_{ET}O_2$, resting pressure of end-tidal O_2. (*From* Fregosi RF, Quan SF, Jackson AC, et al. Ventilatory drive and the apnea-hypopnea index in six-to twelve year old children. BMC Pulm Med 2004;4:4; with permission. Available at: http://www.biomedcentral.com/1471-2466/4/4. Accessed June 23, 2008. Published online 2004 April 29. doi: 10.1186/1471-2466-4-4. Copyright © 2004 Fregosi et al; licensee BioMed Central Ltd. This is an Open Access article: verbatim copying and redistribution of this article are permitted in all media for any purpose, provided this notice is preserved along with the article's original URL.)

Sleep-Disordered Breathing and Oropharyngeal Volume

Whether childhood OSA is associated with a smaller airway was evaluated in another analysis in the TuCASA cohort. MRIs of the pharynx were obtained in 18 awake children 7 to 12 years of age, with OAHI values ranging from 1.81 to 24.2 events/h, to assess the correlation between pharyngeal geometry and soft tissue anatomy and the severity of SDB.[40] The investigators found a positive correlation between the OAHI and the size of tonsils ($r^2 = 0.42$, $P = .024$) and soft palate (proportion of variance of the dependent variable explained [r^2] = 0.33, $P = .049$) and an inverse correlation between the OAHI and the oropharyngeal volume ($r^2 = 0.42$, $P = .038$) and the retropalatal air space (ratio of the retropalatal airway cross-section area to the cross-section area of the soft palate, $r^2 = 0.49$, $P = .001$). As shown in **Fig. 4**, the oropharyngeal volume and the narrowest anterior-posterior oropharyngeal diameter were reduced in the high OAHI group. The high OAHI group had a narrower retropalatal airway where the adenoids, tonsils, and soft palate overlap than the low-OAHI group. The narrow upper airway likely contributes to worse SDB in children who have a high OAHI.

PSYCHOMOTOR VIGILANCE TASK PERFORMANCE

Although the PVT is commonly used as a marker of vigilance in adults, no normative data in children exist. In a TuCASA analysis by Venker and colleagues,[15] normal PVT performance values were derived by analyzing data from a subsample composed of children who had an RDI3% less than one and no parent-reported sleep problems (n = 162). Approximately 51% of this subsample was female. The reaction time (RT) decreased with increasing age, with children 11 years of age (n = 15) having a mean RT of 396.3 milliseconds compared with 721.15 milliseconds in children 6 years of age (n = 27). Boys and girls had

statistically significantly different median RT ($P<.001$). Boys had a shorter median RT (659.4 versus 787.6 ms) and fewer lapses (39.0 versus 58.2) than girls at age 6, but performance on both measures was approximately equal by age 11. The interaction between gender and age was also significant. For boys, mean reciprocal RT (calculated because the distribution of mean RT was positively skewed) is expected to be 2.06 seconds^{-1} at age 6, and is expected to increase by 0.191 seconds^{-1} with each additional year of age. For girls, mean reciprocal RT is expected to be 1.61 seconds^{-1} at age 6, and is expected to increase by 0.274 seconds^{-1} with each additional year of age. The results were not different in Hispanic or Caucasian participants. The median number of total errors was lower for girls than for boys (four versus nine). This improvement in performance among school-aged children is consistent with the neurocognitive and physiologic development taking place during these years.

BEHAVIORAL PROBLEMS ASSOCIATED WITH OVERWEIGHT

Of the 480 sleep studies completed in TuCASA, 402 (83.7%) had complete anthropometric and behavioral data available and constituted the sample for a study assessing the relationships among obesity, SDB, and behavioral problems.[41] Fifty-nine out of these 402 children (~15%) were classified as overweight (at or above the 95th percentile for their age and gender group). The children in the overweight group were slightly older (9.2 versus 8.7 years, $P = .04$) and more likely to be Hispanic (55.9% versus 35.6%, $P<.01$) compared with the non-overweight group. No significant differences existed in gender, RDI0, or parent education between the two groups. Overweight children were more likely to be classified in the clinical range for psychosomatic complaints (OR 2.15, CI 1.02–4.54) on the CPRS-R. The Conners' psychosomatic complaints scale includes items related to headaches, stomach aches in general, stomach aches before school, vague complaints that are not supported by physical illness, and fatigue. However, this difference was not significant when adjusted for SDB.

Overweight children also had a higher probability of being classified within the clinical range for internalizing symptoms (OR 2.23, CI 1.05–4.72), withdrawal (OR 4.69, CI 2.05–10.73), and social problems (OR 3.18, CI 1.53–6.60) on the CBCL. When adjusted for SDB, the probability of clinically relevant withdrawal (OR 3.83, CI 1.59–9.22) and social problems (OR 2.49, CI 1.14–5.44) remained significantly higher for overweight subjects. The

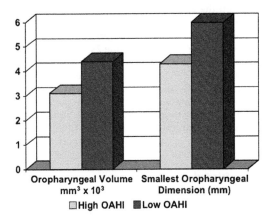

Fig. 4. Oropharyngeal volume ($P<.001$) and the smallest oropharyngeal anterior posterior dimension ($P = .024$) in the high OAHI group (mean OAHI 13.5/h) were reduced in comparison to the low OAHI group (mean OAHI 2.8/h). (*Data from* Fregosi RF, Quan SF, Kaemingk KL, et al. Sleep-disordered breathing, pharyngeal size and soft tissue anatomy in children. J Appl Phys 2003;95:2030–8.)

CBCL withdrawn scale includes items related to inhibition and withdrawal and predicts anxiety and depression.[42] Social scale items are related to social incompetence and being teased and disliked by peers. Overweight children may be bullied and teased by their peers because of their weight, whereas withdrawal may be a secondary to self-conscious behavior or judgment by peers.

SUMMARY

TuCASA is a prospective cohort study of children aged 6 to 12 years that has helped elucidate anatomic and physiologic correlates of SDB and associated clinical outcomes in this age group. The analyses from this epidemiologic study suggest that obesity and SDB are associated with increased behavioral morbidity. Parasomnias, erstwhile considered benign occurrences in children, were shown to be associated with SDB. Furthermore, learning was impaired in children who had PSG-documented SDB. Anatomic and physiologic substudies revealed that children who have SDB have smaller upper airways, increased tonsillar and palatal soft tissue volume, and more collapsible upper airways. Furthermore, SDB may be associated with increased $P_{ET}CO_2$ and depressed hypoxic responsiveness. In the future, results from a 4-year follow-up of the TuCASA cohort will be available, which should result in further information concerning the potential impact of SDB on childhood learning, development, and physiology.

ACKNOWLEDGMENTS

The authors thank Dr. James Goodwin, all the other TuCASA investigators, and the many research staff for their perseverance and dedication to this project, without whom the success of TuCASA would not have occurred.

REFERENCES

1. Gaultier C. Clinical and therapeutic aspects of obstructive sleep apnea syndrome in infants and children. Sleep 1992;15(6 Suppl):S36–8.
2. Guilleminault C. Obstructive sleep apnea. The clinical syndrome and historical perspective. Med Clin North Am 1985;69(6):1187–203.
3. Chervin RD, Archbold KH. Hyperactivity and polysomnographic findings in children evaluated for sleep-disordered breathing. Sleep 2001;24(3):313–20.
4. Gozal D. Sleep-disordered breathing and school performance in children. Pediatrics 1998;102(3 Pt 1):616–20.
5. Owens J, Opipari L, Nobile C, et al. Sleep and daytime behavior in children with obstructive sleep apnea and behavioral sleep disorders. Pediatrics 1998;102(5):1178–84.
6. Hansen DE, Vandenberg B. Neuropsychological features and differential diagnosis of sleep apnea syndrome in children. J Clin Child Psychol 1997;26(3):304–10.
7. Redline S, Tishler PV, Schluchter M, et al. Risk factors for sleep-disordered breathing in children. Associations with obesity, race, and respiratory problems. Am J Respir Crit Care Med 1999;159(5 Pt 1):1527–32.
8. Goodwin JL, Kaemingk KL, Mulvaney SA, et al. Clinical screening of school children for polysomnography to detect sleep-disordered breathing–the Tucson Children's Assessment of Sleep Apnea study (TuCASA). J Clin Sleep Med 2005;1(3):247–54.
9. Redline S, Sanders MH, Lind BK, et al. Methods for obtaining and analyzing unattended polysomnography data for a multicenter study. Sleep Heart Health Research Group. Sleep 1998;21(7):759–67.
10. Rechtschaffen A, Kales A, editors. A manual of standardized terminology, techniques, and scoring system for sleep stages of human subjects. Los Angeles (CA): Brain Information Service/Brain Research Institute, UCLA; 1968.
11. EEG arousals: scoring rules and examples: a preliminary report from the Sleep Disorders Atlas Task Force of the American Sleep Disorders Association. Sleep 1992;15(2):173–84.
12. Conners CK, Sitarenios G, Parker JD, et al. The revised Conners' Parent Rating Scale (CPRS-R): factor structure, reliability, and criterion validity. J Abnorm Child Psychol 1998;26(4):257–68.
13. Achenbach T. Integrative guide for the 1991 CBCL/4-18, YSR, and TRF profiles. Burlington (VT): University of Vermont Department of Psychiatry; 1991.
14. Kaemingk KL, Pasvogel AE, Goodwin JL, et al. Learning in children and sleep disordered breathing: findings of the Tucson Children's Assessment of Sleep Apnea (TuCASA) prospective cohort study. J Int Neuropsychol Soc 2003;9(7):1016–26.
15. Venker CC, Goodwin JL, Roe DJ, et al. Normative psychomotor vigilance task performance in children ages 6 to 11–the Tucson Children's Assessment of Sleep Apnea (TuCASA). Sleep Breath 2007;11(4):217–24.
16. Wechsler abbreviated scale of intelligence. San Antonio (TX): The Psychological Corporation; 1999.
17. Woodcock RW, Johnson MB. Woodcock-Johnson psycho-educational battery–revised. Allen (TX): DLM Teaching Resources; 1989.
18. Talley J. Children's auditory verbal learning test-2. Odessa (FL): Psychological Assessment Resources, Inc; 1993.

19. Goodwin JL, Kaemingk KL, Fregosi RF, et al. Clinical outcomes associated with sleep-disordered breathing in Caucasian and Hispanic children–the Tucson Children's Assessment of Sleep Apnea study (TuCASA). Sleep 2003;26(5):587–91.

20. Redline S, Budhiraja R, Kapur V, et al. The scoring of respiratory events in sleep: reliability and validity. J Clin Sleep Med 2007;3(2):169–200.

21. Budhiraja R, Goodwin JL, Parthasarathy S, et al. Comparison of nasal pressure transducer and thermistor for detection of respiratory events during polysomnography in children. Sleep 2005;28(9): 1117–21.

22. Budhiraja R, Sharief I, Quan SF. Sleep disordered breathing and hypertension. J Clin Sleep Med 2005;1(4):401–4.

23. Budhiraja R, Quan SF. Sleep-disordered breathing and cardiovascular health. Curr Opin Pulm Med 2005;11(6):501–6.

24. Update on the 1987 Task Force Report on High Blood Pressure in Children and Adolescents: a working group report from the National High Blood Pressure Education Program. National High Blood Pressure Education Program Working Group on Hypertension Control in Children and Adolescents. Pediatrics 1996;98(4 Pt 1):649–58.

25. Enright PL, Goodwin JL, Sherrill DL, et al. Blood pressure elevation associated with sleep-related breathing disorder in a community sample of white and Hispanic children: the Tucson Children's Assessment of Sleep Apnea study. Arch Pediatr Adolesc Med 2003;157(9):901–4.

26. Rosner B, Prineas R, Loggie J, et al. Percentiles for body mass index in U.S. children 5 to 17 years of age. J Pediatr 1998;132(2):211–22.

27. Rosner B, Prineas RJ, Loggie JM, et al. Blood pressure nomograms for children and adolescents, by height, sex, and age, in the United States. J Pediatr 1993;123(6):871–86.

28. Marcus CL, Greene MG, Carroll JL. Blood pressure in children with obstructive sleep apnea. Am J Respir Crit Care Med 1998;157(4 Pt 1):1098–103.

29. Budhiraja R, Parthasarathy S, Quan SF. Endothelial dysfunction in obstructive sleep apnea. J Clin Sleep Med 2007;3(4):409–15.

30. Mulvaney SA, Goodwin JL, Morgan WJ, et al. Behavior problems associated with sleep disordered breathing in school-aged children–the Tucson Children's Assessment of Sleep Apnea study. J Pediatr Psychol 2006;31(3):322–30.

31. Gau SF, Soong WT. Psychiatric comorbidity of adolescents with sleep terrors or sleepwalking: a case-control study. Aust N Z J Psychiatry 1999;33(5): 734–9.

32. Owens J, Spirito A, Nobile C, et al. Incidence of parasomnias in children with obstructive sleep apnea. Sleep 1997;20(12):1193–6.

33. Mahowald MW, Rosen GM. Parasomnias in children. Pediatrician 1990;17(1):21–31.

34. Goodwin JL, Kaemingk KL, Fregosi RF, et al. Parasomnias and sleep disordered breathing in Caucasian and Hispanic children - the Tucson Children's Assessment of Sleep Apnea study. BMC Med 2004;2:14.

35. Guilleminault C, Palombini L, Pelayo R, et al. Sleepwalking and sleep terrors in prepubertal children: what triggers them? Pediatrics Jan 2003;111(1): e17–25.

36. Fregosi RF, Quan SF, Jackson AC, et al. Ventilatory drive and the apnea-hypopnea index in six-to-twelve year old children. BMC Pulm Med 2004;4:4.

37. Kerbl R, Zotter H, Schenkeli R, et al. Persistent hypercapnia in children after treatment of obstructive sleep apnea syndrome by adenotonsillectomy. Wien Klin Wochenschr 2001;113(7–8):229–34.

38. Marcus CL, Katz ES, Lutz J, et al. Upper airway dynamic responses in children with the obstructive sleep apnea syndrome. Pediatr Res 2005;57(1): 99–107.

39. Fregosi RF, Quan SF, Morgan WL, et al. Pharyngeal critical pressure in children with mild sleep-disordered breathing. J Appl Phys 2006;101(3):734–9.

40. Fregosi RF, Quan SF, Kaemingk KL, et al. Sleep-disordered breathing, pharyngeal size and soft tissue anatomy in children. J Appl Phys 2003;95(5): 2030–8.

41. Mulvaney SA, Kaemingk KL, Goodwin JL, et al. Parent-rated behavior problems associated with overweight before and after controlling for sleep disordered breathing. BMC Pediatr 2006;6:34.

42. Kasius MC, Ferdinand RF, van den Berg H, et al. Associations between different diagnostic approaches for child and adolescent psychopathology. J Child Psychol Psychiatry 1997;38(6):625–32.

Sleep Problems in Children with Autism, ADHD, Anxiety, Depression, Acquired Brain Injury, and Typical Development

Susan Dickerson Mayes, PhD[a],*, Susan Calhoun, PhD[b],
Edward O. Bixler, PhD[b], Alexandros N. Vgontzas, MD[b]

KEYWORDS

- Sleep • Autism • ADHD • Anxiety
- Depression • Brain injury

AUTISM AND SLEEP

More than half of parents of children with autism report a sleep disturbance in their children.[1–9] Compared with normal controls, parents note that children who have autism have more trouble falling asleep, wake more during the night, awake earlier in the morning, have greater sleep walking and talking and bed wetting, and sleep less.[1,5,7,10–12] Objective sleep laboratory polysomnographic (PSG) studies also show sleep disturbances in children who have autism, including REM sleep abnormalities[13,14] and decreased sleep duration.[15] Children who have autism and sleep problems have more severe autistic symptoms (specifically social and affective problems) than children who have autism and do not have sleep problems.[16]

ANXIETY, DEPRESSION, AND SLEEP

Parent and self-reported sleep problems are prevalent in children with depression[2,17–20] and anxiety disorders.[19–23] Parent-reported sleep problems also correlate significantly with parent ratings of anxiety and depression.[24] Some PSG studies show sleep abnormalities in children with depression, such as prolonged sleep latency,[25] reduced REM movement latencies,[26] decreased sleep efficiency and delayed sleep onset,[27] and electroencephalographic rhythm abnormalities.[28] In contrast, two other electroencephalographic sleep studies did not demonstrate sleep problems in children with depression.[17,29]

MENTAL RETARDATION, NEUROLOGIC CONDITIONS, AND SLEEP

Most parents of children with mental retardation report sleep problems in their children,[30–33] with sleep problems occurring at two to four times the normal frequency.[33,34] PSG studies in children who have Down syndrome show decreased REM sleep[13] and increased occurrence of sleep-disordered

This study was supported by the NHLBI Grant RO1-HL63722, the General Clinical Research Center Grants MO1-RR10732 and CO6-RR016499, Autism Speaks, Organization for Autism Research, and the Children's Miracle Network.

[a] Department of Psychiatry, Milton S. Hershey Medical Center, Penn State College of Medicine, 500 University Drive, Hershey, PA 17033, USA

[b] Department of Psychiatry, Sleep Research and Treatment Center, Penn State College of Medicine, H073, 500 University Drive, Hershey, PA 17033, USA

* Corresponding author.
E-mail address: smayes@psu.edu (S.D. Mayes).

Sleep Med Clin 4 (2009) 19–25
doi:10.1016/j.jsmc.2008.12.004
1556-407X/08/$ – see front matter

breathing.[35] Subjective and objective studies show high frequencies of sleep problems in children with neurologic impairments.[36] For example, sleep problems are common in children with epilepsy and cerebral palsy,[32,37,38] traumatic brain injury,[39,40] chromosomal disorders,[36,41] brain malformations,[36] and brain damage related to intraventricular hemorrhage or perinatal asphyxia.[41]

ADHD AND SLEEP

Many children with ADHD have parent-reported sleep problems.[42–47] Children with ADHD also have greater movements during sleep than children without ADHD.[44,48–50] PSG sleep data do not show differences between children with ADHD and controls in sleep latency and efficiency, nighttime awakenings, and sleep stages, however.[50–57] Data for sleep-disordered breathing are inconsistent. Children with ADHD had a higher apnea-hypopnea index than controls in two studies[52,55] but not in another study.[51] Similarly, ratings of ADHD symptoms did not differ between children with and without sleep-disordered breathing in another study.[58]

Our recent study of children with ADHD and community control children[59] showed that daytime sleepiness was not significantly correlated with sleeping less than normal but was associated with sleeping more than normal. Children who had longer sleep durations also had greater daytime sleepiness, which suggested that children who were sleepier during the day were also sleepier at night. This finding is contrary to the common belief that if children sleep less at night, they are sleepier during the day. This may be the case for some children but was not true for our large samples of children with ADHD ($n = 681$) and typical development ($n = 135$). Other ADHD studies also found that daytime sleepiness was not related to parent report of sleep problems[60] or objective PSG measures of sleep problems.[57] These findings are consistent with a PSG study in adults that showed that sleepiness in obese patients with and without sleep apnea was not related to disturbed sleep.[61]

ADHD AND SLEEP: MEDIATING FACTORS
ADHD Subtype

By definition, children with ADHD-combined type (ADHD-C) have an attention deficit, impulsivity, and hyperactivity, whereas children with ADHD-inattentive type (ADHD-I) have only an attention deficit without impulsivity and hyperactivity.[62] In our parent-report study of 135 community control children and 681 children with ADHD-C or ADHD-I,

children with ADHD-I had significantly fewer sleep problems than children with ADHD-C and they did not differ from typical controls.[59] Children with ADHD-I experienced greater daytime sleepiness than children with ADHD-C, which suggested a neurophysiologic underarousal in ADHD-I. Sluggish cognitive tempo, slow processing speed, underarousal, and underactivity are associated with ADHD-I more often than with ADHD-C.[63–69] ADHD-I may be characterized by global physiologic underarousal that affects all areas of functioning, including activity level, cognitive tempo, and sleep. Children with ADHD-C in our study slept less than normal but did not differ from controls on daytime sleepiness. Children with ADHD-C may have intrinsically high levels of energy, regardless of sleep duration. Research also shows that children with ADHD-C have increased movement during sleep, whereas children with ADHD-I do not.[44] This finding suggests that ADHD-C may be a "24-hour disorder" for some children.[49]

Studies indicate that sleep is a potentially important dimension differentiating ADHD-C and ADHD-I subtypes. The two subtypes differ not only in ADHD symptoms but also physiologically, as indicated by differences in their nighttime sleep and daytime alertness. Objective PSG studies show better sleep efficiency and less fragmented sleep in children with ADHD-I than ADHD-C.[70] Children with ADHD-I do not have increased movement during sleep, whereas children with ADHD-C do.[44] Children with ADHD-I have fewer parent-reported sleep problems than children with ADHD-C,[59] and children with ADHD-I have greater parent-reported daytime sleepiness than children with ADHD-C.[59,60] Daytime sleepiness determined by multiple sleep latency tests is also greater in children with ADHD-I than in children with ADHD-C.[57] These findings point to the critical need to differentiate between ADHD-C and ADHD-I subtypes in sleep research studies, because combining the two types (which most studies do) confounds research findings.

ADHD Severity

Correlations between parent ratings of sleep problems and ADHD symptoms are significant for children with ADHD.[59] This relationship often has been interpreted as indicating that sleep problems cause ADHD-like symptoms.[62] It is reasonable to hypothesize that sleep problems have a negative impact on daytime functioning for some children; however, this does not mean that sleep problems are a primary cause of attention deficit or hyperactivity. Existing studies are purely correlational (not causal). The association may not be unidirectional (ie, ADHD may cause sleep problems) or causal (ie, sleep problems and ADHD may be comorbid and have a common neurophysiologic etiology, explaining the relationship between the two).

ADHD Comorbidity

Little has been published on the relationship between comorbidity in ADHD and sleep problems.[49] In one study,[44] ADHD in combination with oppositional-defiant disorder was associated with resistance to going to bed and resistance to waking in the morning. In the same study, ADHD with anxiety was significantly correlated with increased movement during sleep. Comorbid depression was linked with greater self-report of sleep problems in adolescents with ADHD in another study.[71] In our study,[59] total sleep problems scores were significantly greater in children with ADHD when anxiety or depression was present than when anxiety or depression was absent. In contrast, sleep problems did not differ significantly between children with ADHD who had oppositional-defiant disorder versus children with ADHD who did not.

ADHD Medication

In controlled studies, sleep latency did not differ between children with ADHD on methylphenidate versus placebo,[72,73] but total sleep duration was shorter with methylphenidate than placebo.[73] Using subjective reports, medicated versus unmedicated children with ADHD did not differ in sleep disturbance in one study,[42] but medicated children had greater sleep problems in other studies.[47,71] Medicated children have more severe ADHD symptoms than nonmedicated children, however, which have not been controlled in subjective sleep studies.[71] When ADHD severity was controlled in a recent study,[59] children on medication versus children not on medication did not differ in most parent-reported sleep problems, including difficulty falling asleep, waking during the night, restlessness during sleep, nightmares, walking or talking in sleep, bed wetting, waking too early, and sleeping less than normal. Children with ADHD on medication had significantly greater difficulty falling asleep than children not on medication, however.

COMPARATIVE ANALYSIS OF SLEEP PROBLEMS IN CLINICAL AND TYPICAL CHILDREN

This section reports data for 650 clinical children and 135 community control children aged 6 to 16 years in a study that compared the frequency

and type of parent-reported sleep problems in children with autism, ADHD-C, ADHD-I, anxiety, depression, acquired brain injury (eg, closed head injury or spina bifida with hydrocephalus), and typical development.[5] No previous study has investigated the relative frequency of sleep problems in children with these diagnoses. The 650 clinical children were consecutive referrals to our child psychiatry clinic and had normal intelligence (WISC-III or WISC-IV IQ $\geq$ 80) and a confirmatory diagnosis by another psychologist or physician. The control sample comprised 135 elementary school children without psychiatric diagnoses or learning disorders who were subjects in a general population epidemiologic study of sleep disorders in children. Parents rated their children on a 4-point scale from "not at all a problem" to "very often a problem" on the 165 items on the Pediatric Behavior Scale (PBS).[74] The PBS yields a total sleep problems T-score and scores on 10 sleep items: (1) having difficulty falling asleep, (2) waking often during the night, (3) being restless during sleep, (4) having nightmares, (5) walking or talking in sleep, (6) wetting bed, (7) waking too early, (8) sleeping less than most children, (9) sleeping more than most children, and (10) being sleepy during the day.

Overall sleep problems T-scores were significantly higher for children with autism ($T = 66$) than for all other groups, including ADHD-C ($T = 61$), anxiety or depression ($T = 61$), brain injury ($T = 57$), normal controls ($T = 57$), and ADHD-I ($T = 55$), $F = 7.3$, $P < .0001$, pairwise $t = 2.1$ to 5.6, $P < .05$. Children with ADHD-C had significantly greater sleep problems T-scores than children with ADHD-I ($t = 3.4$, $P = .001$) and controls ($t = 2.1$, $P = .03$). All other comparisons were nonsignificant, except that children with ADHD-I had lower sleep problems T-scores than children with anxiety or depression ($t = 2.1$, $P = .03$).

The percentages of children whose mothers rated each type of sleep problem as "sometimes" to "very often" a problem are reported in **Table 1**. Children with autism had the highest mean sleep problems scores on seven of the eight nighttime sleep problems. They had significantly higher scores than all other groups on difficulty falling asleep, waking early, and sleeping less than normal ($t = 2.3$ to 8.0, $P < .02$) and higher scores on bed wetting than all other groups ($t = 2.3$ to 4.7, $P < .03$), except brain injury ($t = 1.8$, $P = .08$).

Children with ADHD-C had greater difficulty falling asleep, slept less, and had more bed wetting than controls ($t = 2.9$ to 3.3, $P < .005$), and they had less daytime sleepiness than children with autism, ADHD-I, and anxiety or depression ($t = 2.0$ to 4.2, $P < .05$). Children with anxiety or

Table 1
Percentage of children with each type of sleep problem

	Controls	ADHD-I	ADHD-C	Autism	Anxiety/Depression	Brain Injury
Sleeps more than normal	16	17	13	13	27	21
Sleeps less than normal	12	19	24	45	15	21
Difficulty falling asleep	41	40	48	61	55	39
Restless during sleep	48	34	47	51	48	36
Wakes often	36	24	38	39	38	24
Nightmares	44	26	42	52	40	30
Walks or talks in sleep	35	28	36	33	30	30
Wets bed	10	10	21	29	7	21
Wakes too early	24	22	31	42	17	21
Daytime sleepiness	12	24	12	26	30	21

depression slept more than all other groups ($t = 2.3$ to 2.7, $P < .03$) except for children with brain injury ($t = 1.5$, $P = .14$). Children with anxiety or depression also had greater daytime sleepiness than children with ADHD-C and controls ($t = 2.4$ and 2.4, $P = .02$). Children with ADHD-I had significantly less restlessness during sleep, less waking during the night, and fewer nightmares than children with autism, ADHD-C, and anxiety or depression ($t = 2.0$ to 4.2, $P < .05$). Controls had less daytime sleepiness than children with autism, ADHD-I, and anxiety or depression ($t = 2.0$ to 3.9, $P < .05$). Children with brain injury had sleep problems scores in the midrange for all types of sleep problems and differed significantly only from children with autism on a few of the sleep problems scores.

Restlessness during sleep and difficulty falling asleep were the most common sleep problems for all groups, yielding significantly higher mean scores than most other types of sleep problems. In contrast, bed wetting, sleeping more than normal, and daytime sleepiness were the least common problems, with mean scores significantly lower than most other sleep problems ($F = 21.6$ to 346.2, $P < .0001$).

SUMMARY AND IMPLICATIONS

A comparative analysis of the frequency and type of parent-reported sleep problems in children with clinical disorders and community controls[5] showed that (1) children with anxiety or depression slept more than children with autism, ADHD-C, ADHD-I, acquired brain injury, and typical development; (2) children with autism had significantly more difficulty falling asleep, woke earlier, slept less, and had more bed wetting than children in the other diagnostic groups; (3) children with

ADHD-I had fewer sleep problems than the other clinical groups but had more daytime sleepiness than typical controls; (4) children with ADHD-C had significantly more sleep problems than controls; (5) controls and children with ADHD-C had the least daytime sleepiness, and (6) children with brain injury had sleep problems scores that were in the midrange compared with all other groups.

Overall, children with autism and ADHD-C had the highest frequency of parent-reported sleep problems, with more than half of these children having at least one type of sleep problem. Medical practitioners and clinicians need to be aware of the risk of sleep problems in children with autism and ADHD-C and should screen routinely for sleep problems in these children and recommend intervention as needed. Evidence-based treatments are available to reduce sleep problems in children. Blind placebo-controlled studies showed that melatonin improves sleep in children with ADHD,[75,76] autism,[77] and epilepsy,[78] and a multiple baseline study demonstrated the effectiveness of behavior therapy in reducing sleep problems in children with autism.[79]

REFERENCES

1. Hering E, Epstein R, Elroy S, et al. Sleep patterns in autistic children. J Autism Dev Disord 2003;29:143–7.
2. Ivanenko A, Crabtree VM, Gozal D. Sleep in children with psychiatric disorders. Pediatr Clin North Am 2004;51:51–68.
3. Liu X, Hubbard JA, Fabes RA, et al. Sleep disturbances and correlates of children with autism spectrum disorders. Child Psychiatry Hum Dev 2006;37:179–91.

4. Mayes SD, Calhoun SL. Symptoms of autism in young children and correspondence with the DSM. Infants Young Child 1999;12:90–7.

5. Mayes SD, Calhoun SL, Bixler EO, et al. Sleep disorders in clinical and typical children. Annual Meeting of the Penn State Sleep Disorders Medicine Symposium, Hershey, PA, November 2, 2007.

6. Polimeni MA, Richdale AL, Francis AJ. A survey of sleep problems in autism, Asperger's disorder and typically developing children. J Intellect Disabil Res 2005;49:260–8.

7. Richdale A, Prior MR. The sleep/wake rhythm in children with autism. Eur Child Adolesc Psychiatry 1995;4:175–86.

8. Wiggs L, Stores G. Sleep patterns and sleep disorders in children with autistic spectrum disorders: insights using parent report and actigraphy. Dev Med Child Neurol 2004;46:372–80.

9. Williams PG, Sears LL, Allard A. Sleep problems in children with autism. J Sleep Res 2004;13:265–8.

10. Allik H, Larsson JO, Smedje H. Sleep patterns of school-age children with Asperger syndrome or high-functioning autism. J Autism Dev Disord 2006; 36:585–95.

11. Couturier JL, Speechley KN, Steele M, et al. Parental perception of sleep problems in children of normal intelligence with pervasive developmental disorders: prevalence, severity, and pattern. J Am Acad Child Adolesc Psychiatry 2005;44:815–22.

12. Patzold LM, Richdale AL, Tonge BJ. An investigation into sleep characteristics of children with autism and Asperger's disorder. J Paediatr Child Health 1998; 34:528–33.

13. Diomedi M, Curatolo P, Scalise A, et al. Sleep abnormalities in mentally retarded autistic subjects: Down's syndrome with mental retardation and normal subjects. Brain Dev 1999;21:548–53.

14. Thirumalai SS, Shubin RA, Robinson R. Rapid eye movement sleep behavior disorder in children with autism. J Child Neurol 2002;17:173–8.

15. Elia M, Ferri R, Musumeci SA, et al. Sleep in subjects with autistic disorder: a neurophysiological and psychological study. Brain Dev 2000;22:88–92.

16. Malow BA, Marzec ML, McGrew SG, et al. Characterizing sleep in children with autism spectrum disorders: a multidimensional approach. Sleep 2006;29:1563–71.

17. Bertocci MA, Dahl RE, Williamson DE, et al. Subjective sleep complaints in pediatric depression: a controlled study and comparison with EEG measures of sleep and waking. J Am Acad Child Adolesc Psychiatry 2005;44:1158–66.

18. Dahl RE, Lewin DS. Sleep and depression. In: Stores G, Wiggs L, editors. Sleep disturbance in children and adolescents with disorders of development: its significance and management. Oxford, England: Cambridge University Press; 2001. p. 161–8.

19. Mindell JA, Owens JA, Carskadon MA. Developmental features of sleep. Child Adolesc Psychiatr Clin N Am 1999;8:695–725.

20. Stores G, Wiggs L. Children at high risk of sleep disturbance. In: Stores G, editor. A clinical guide to sleep disorders in children and adolescents. Oxford, England: Cambridge University Press; 2001. p. 15–24.

21. Alfano CA, Beidel DC, Turner SM, et al. Preliminary evidence for sleep complaints among children referred for anxiety. Sleep Med 2006;7:467–73.

22. Garland EJ. Sleep disturbances in anxious children. In: Stores G, Wiggs L, editors. Sleep disturbance in children and adolescents with disorders of development: its significance and management. Oxford, England: Cambridge University Press; 2001. p. 155–60.

23. Kendall PC, Pimentel SS. On the physiological symptom constellation in youth with generalized anxiety disorder (GAD). J Anxiety Disord 2003;17: 211–21.

24. Johnson EO, Chilcoat HD, Breslau N. Trouble sleeping and anxiety/depression in childhood. Psychiatry Res 2000;94:93–102.

25. Dahl RE, Ryan ND, Matty MK, et al. Sleep onset abnormalities in depressed adolescents. Biol Psychiatry 1996;39:400–10.

26. Emslie GJ, Rush AJ, Weinberg WA, et al. Children with major depression show reduced rapid eye movement latencies. Arch Gen Psychiatry 1990;7: 119–24.

27. Emslie GJ, Armitage R, Weinberg WA, et al. Sleep polysomnography as a predictor of recurrence in children and adolescents with major depressive disorder. Int J Neuropsychopharmacol 2001;4: 159–68.

28. Armitage R, Emsilie GJ, Hoffmann RF, et al. Ultradian rhythms and temporal coherence in sleep EEG in depressed children and adolescents. Biol Psychiatry 2000;47:338–50.

29. Dahl RE, Puig-Antich J, Ryan ND, et al. EEG sleep in adolescents with major depression: the role of suicidality and inpatient status. J Affect Disord 1990;19: 63–75.

30. Hayashi E, Katada A. Sleep in persons with intellectual disabilities: a questionnaire survey. Japanese Journal of Special Education 2002;39:91–101.

31. Piazza CC, Fisher WW, Kahng SW. Sleep patterns in children and young adults with mental retardation and severe behavior disorders. Dev Med Child Neurol 1996;38:335–44.

32. Quine L. Sleep problems in children with mental handicap. J Ment Defic Res 1991;35:269–90.

33. Richdale A, Francis A, Gavidia-Payne S, et al. Stress, behaviour, and sleep problems in children with an intellectual disability. J Intellect Dev Disabil 2000;25:147–61.

34. Quine L. Sleep problems in primary school children: comparison between mainstream and special school children. Child Care Health Dev 2000;27: 201–21.

35. Miguel-Diez J, Villa-Asensi JR, Alvarez-Sala JL. Prevalence of sleep-disordered breathing in children with Down syndrome: polygraphic findings in 108 children. Sleep 2003;26:1006–9.

36. Grigg-Damberger M. Neurologic disorders masquerading as pediatric sleep problems. Pediatr Clin North Am 2004;51:89–115.

37. Becker DA, Fennell EB, Carney PR. Sleep disturbance in children with epilepsy. Epilepsy Behav 2003;4:651–8.

38. Zucconi M, Bruni O. Sleep disorders in children with neurologic diseases. Semin Pediatr Neurol 2001;8: 258–75.

39. Bandla H, Splaingard M. Sleep problems in children with common medical disorders. Pediatr Clin North Am 2004;51:203–27.

40. Patten SB, Lauderdale MW. Delayed sleep phase disorder after traumatic brain injury. J Am Acad Child Adolesc Psychiatry 1992;31:100–2.

41. Halpern LF, MacLena WE, Baumeister AA. Infant sleep-wake characteristics: relation to neurological status and the prediction of developmental outcome. Dev Rev 1995;15:255–91.

42. Ball JD, Tiernan M, Janusz J, et al. Sleep patterns among children with attention-deficit hyperactivity disorder: a reexamination of parent perceptions. J Pediatr Psychol 1997;22:389–98.

43. Chervin RD, Dillon JE, Bassetti C, et al. Symptoms of sleep disorders, inattention, and hyperactivity in children. Sleep 1997;20:1185–92.

44. Corkum P, Moldofsky H, Hogg-Johnson S, et al. Sleep problems in children with attention-deficit/hyperactivity disorder: impact of subtype, comorbidity, and stimulant medication. J Am Acad Child Adolesc Psychiatry 1999;38:1285–93.

45. Corkum P, Tannock R, Moldofsky H, et al. Actigraphy and parental ratings of sleep in children with attention-deficit/hyperactivity disorder (ADHD). Sleep 2001;24:303–12.

46. Ring A, Stein D, Barak Y, et al. Sleep disturbances in children with attention-deficit/hyperactivity disorder: a comparative study. J Learn Disabil 1998;31:572–8.

47. Stein MA. Unravelling sleep problems in treated and untreated children with ADHD. J Child Adolesc Psychopharmacol 1999;9:157–68.

48. Corkum P, Tannock R, Moldofsky H. Sleep disturbance in children with attention-deficit/hyperactivity disorder. J Am Acad Child Adolesc Psychiatry 1998;37:637–46.

49. Cortese S, Konofal E, Yareman N, et al. Sleep and alertness in children with attention-deficit/hyperactivity disorder: a systematic review of the literature. Sleep 2006;29:504–11.

50. Konofal E, Lecendreux M, Bouvard MP, et al. High levels of nocturnal activity in children with attention-deficit hyperactivity disorder: a video analysis. Psychiatry Clin Neurosci 2001;55:97–103.

51. Cooper J, Tyler L, Wallace I, et al. No evidence of sleep apnea in children with attention deficit hyperactivity disorder. Clin Pediatr 2001;43:609–14.

52. Golan N, Shahar E, Ravid S, et al. Sleep disorders and daytime sleepiness in children with attention-deficit/hyperactivity disorder. Sleep 2004;27:261–6.

53. Gruber R, Sadeh A. Sleep and neurobehavioral functioning in boys with attention-deficit/hyperactivity disorder and no reported breathing problems. Sleep 2004;27:267–73.

54. Gruber R, Sadeh A, Raviv A. Instability of sleep patterns in children with attention-deficit/hyperactivity disorder. J Am Acad Child Adolesc Psychiatry 2000;39:495–501.

55. Huang YS, Chen NH, Li HY, et al. Sleep disorders in Taiwanese children with attention deficit/hyperactivity disorder. J Sleep Res 2004;13:269–77.

56. Kirov R, Kinkelbur J, Heipke S, et al. Is there a specific polysomnographic sleep pattern in children with attention deficit/hyperactivity disorder? J Sleep Res 2004;13:87–93.

57. Lecendrueux M, Konofal E, Bouvard M, et al. Sleep and alertness in children with ADHD. J Child Psychol Psychiatry 2000;41:803–12.

58. Chervin RD, Archbold KH. Hyperactivity and polysomnographic findings in children evaluated for sleep-disordered breathing. Sleep 2001;24: 313–20.

59. Mayes SD, Calhoun SL, Bixler EO, et al. ADHD subtypes and comorbid anxiety, depression, and oppositional-defiant disorder: differences in sleep problems. J Pediatr Psychol, in press.

60. LeBourgeois MK, Avis K, Mixon M, et al. Snoring, sleep quality, and sleepiness across attention-deficit/hyperactivity disorder subtypes. Sleep 2004; 27:520–5.

61. Vgontzas AN, Tan TL, Bixler EO, et al. Obesity without sleep apnea is associated with daytime sleepiness. Arch Intern Med 1998;158:1333–7.

62. American Psychiatric Association. Diagnostic and statistical manual of mental disorders. 4th edition, text revision. Washington, DC: Author; 2000.

63. Barkley RA, DuPaul GJ, McMurray MB. Comprehensive evaluation of attention deficit disorder with and without hyperactivity as defined by research criteria. J Consult Clin Psychol 1990;58:775–89.

64. Barkley RA, Grodzinsky G, DuPaul GJ. Frontal lobe functions in attention deficit disorder with and without hyperactivity: a review and research report. J Abnorm Child Psychol 1992;20:163–88.

65. Calhoun SL, Mayes SD. Processing speed in children with clinical disorders. Psychol Sch 2005;42: 333–43.

66. Cantwell DP, Baker L. Attention deficit disorder with and without hyperactivity: a review and comparison of matched groups. J Am Acad Child Adolesc Psychiatry 1992;31:432–8.

67. Goodyear P, Hynd GW. Attention-deficit disorder with and without hyperactivity: behavioral and neuropsychological differentiation. J Clin Child Psychol 1992;21:273–305.

68. Hartman CA, Willcutt EG, Rhee SH, et al. The relation between sluggish cognitive tempo and DSM-IV ADHD. J Abnorm Child Psychol 2004;32:491–503.

69. Stanford LD, Hynd GW. Congruence of behavioral symptomatology in children with ADD/H, ADD/WO, and learning disabilities. J Learn Disabil 1994;27:243–53.

70. Ramos Platon MJ, Vela Bueno A, Espinar Sierra J, et al. Hypnopolygraphic alternations in attention deficit disorder (ADD) children. Int J Dev Neurosci 1990;53:87–101.

71. Stein D, Pat-Horenczyk R, Blank S, et al. Sleep disturbances in adolescents with symptoms of attention-deficit/hyperactivity disorder. J Learn Disabil 2002;35:268–75.

72. Kent JD, Blader JC, Koplewicz HS, et al. Effects of late-afternoon methylphenidate administration on behavior and sleep in attention-deficit hyperactivity disorder. Pediatrics 1995;96:320–5.

73. Tirosh E, Sadeh A, Munvez R, et al. Effects of methylphenidate on sleep in children with attention-deficit hyperactivity disorder. Am J Dis Child 1993;147:1313–5.

74. Lindgren SD, Koeppl GK. Assessing child behavior problems in a medical setting: development of the pediatric behavior scale. In: Prinz RJ, editor. Advances in behavioral assessment of children and families. Greenwich (CT): JAI; 1987. p. 57–90.

75. van der Heijden KB, Smits MG, van Someren EJ, et al. Effect of melatonin on sleep, behavior, and cognition in ADHD and chronic sleep-onset insomnia. J Am Acad Child Adolesc Psychiatry 2007;6:233–41.

76. Weiss MD, Wasdell MB, Bomben MM, et al. Sleep hygiene and melatonin treatment for children and adolescents with ADHD and initial insomnia. J Am Acad Child Adolesc Psychiatry 2006;45:512–9.

77. Garstang J, Wallis M. Randomized controlled trial of melatonin for children with autistic spectrum disorders and sleep problems. Child Care Health Dev 2006;32:585–9.

78. Gupta M, Aneja S, Kohli K. Add-on melatonin improves sleep behavior in children with epilepsy: randomized, double-blind, placebo-controlled trial. J Child Neurol 2005;20:112–5.

79. Weiskop S, Richdale A, Matthews J. Behavioural treatment to reduce sleep problems in children with autism or fragile x syndrome. Dev Med Child Neurol 2005;47:94–104.

Cardiac Autonomic Modulation and Sleep-Disordered Breathing in Children

Duanping Liao, MD, PhD[a],*, Jiahao Liu, MD[a],
Alexandros N. Vgontzas, MD[b], Sol Rodriguez-Colon, MS[a],
Susan Calhoun, PhD[b], Xian Li, MD, MS[a], Edward O. Bixler, PhD[b]

KEYWORDS

- Sleep-disordered breathing • Heart rate variability
- Blood pressure • Population-based study • Obesity
- Sleep stages • Children

It is well known that an episode of apnea is accompanied by a typical pattern of heart rate fluctuations (ie, bradycardia during the apneic phase and tachycardia at the restoration of breathing). Several studies in adults have shown that SDB is associated significantly with lower HRV, indicating impaired cardiac autonomic modulation, in persons who have apnea.[1–4] In the cardiac disease literature, analysis of beat-to-beat HRV has emerged as a clinically and epidemiologically useful noninvasive method to assess cardiac autonomic activity quantitatively.[5–21] Most importantly, lower HRV has been associated consistently with the risk of incident cardiovascular disease.[8–11,19,20,22–24] Little is known, however, about the impact of SDB on cardiac autonomic modulation in children. This article summarizes the authors' current application of HRV analysis in the population-based study of cardiac autonomic modulation in young children.

SLEEP-DISORDERED BREATHING IN CHILDREN

SDB is considered an important cause of morbidity in children and is potentially a major public health problem.[25–30] The understanding of the clinical significance of SDB, especially in children, is limited. Initially, children who had SDB were recognized only after they developed life-threatening problems such as cor pulmonale or growth failure.[29] Today early recognition of SDB is facilitated by polysomnography, but the ability to diagnose milder forms of SDB in children has not been accompanied by any clear understanding of the clinical risk of these milder forms. Thus, it is unclear whether treatment should be prescribed for the milder forms of this disorder or, if so, which treatment should be prescribed. Based on limited data, it was estimated that approximately 10% of children snore during sleep every night or most nights.[31–34] Approximately 1% to 3% of school-aged children are thought to have obstructive sleep apnea, the most severe form of SDB.[35–43] SDB seems to occur equally in boys and girls[32–44] and may be more common in blacks[39,45] and Hispanics.[46] Some data suggested that SDB was associated with a family history[39,47–49] and with environmental exposure to tobacco smoke.[33,35,38,39,50] Enlarged tonsils

The authors have received support from grants NIH R21 HL087858-01, R01 HL63772, M01 RR010732, C06 RR016499.

[a] Department of Public Health Sciences, Pennsylvania State University College of Medicine, 600 Centerview Dr., Suite 2200, A210 Hershey, PA 17033, USA

[b] Department of Psychiatry, Sleep Research and Treatment Center, Penn State College of Medicine, H073, 500 University Drive, Hershey, PA 17033, USA

* Corresponding author.

E-mail address: dliao@psu.edu (D. Liao).

and adenoids often are said to be the cause of SDB[51–53] in children, but adenotonsillar hypertrophy alone is not sufficient to produce sleep apnea, and the severity of sleep apnea does not correlate with the degree of adenotonsillar enlargement.[51] Further, some persons who have undergone adenotonsillectomy for sleep apnea have developed recurrent symptoms.[28] Recently, pulmonary symptoms (eg, sinus problems, persistent wheeze) have been shown to be associated with SDB in children.[39]

A growing body of clinically derived data suggests that SDB in children is associated with severe consequences. The pediatric literature is replete with reports of children who have obstructive sleep apnea presenting with cardiovascular disorders (eg, cor pulmonale or congestive heart failure).[43,44,54–58] Data regarding the association with hypertension are conflicting, however. For example, in a series of 50 cases, systemic hypertension was found in 10% of patients, all of whom were older than 10 years.[44] More recently, obesity, sleep efficiency, and SDB were observed to be associated independently with elevated blood pressure in a sample of 239 children aged 6 to 11 years.[59] It is clear that sleep apnea has cardiovascular consequences, but the nature and extent of these consequences, particularly in milder forms of apnea, is unknown.

Poor somatic growth or failure to thrive commonly has been associated with SDB in children. In earlier studies based primarily on severe sleep apnea, between 27% and 69% of children were found to have growth failure.[43,44,60–62] More recently poor weight gain has been associated with milder cases of SDB,[40,63] and severe cases of sleep apnea also have been shown to affect growth without full-blown failure to thrive.[64] Improvement in somatic growth following adenotonsillectomy in children suspected of having sleep apnea has been reported.[43,54,65–67] In one study, 52% of 29 children studied were failing to thrive.[66] Eighty-seven percent of those failing to thrive preoperatively showed improved weight gain postoperatively. Growth hormone deficiency has been implicated in sleep fragmentation,[68] but results are conflicting, and no systematic evaluation has been completed.

Cognitive and behavioral abnormalities, including academic performance, learning and memory disabilities, attention disorders, developmental delay, hyperactivity, aggression, and withdrawn behavior, have been associated with sleep apnea in children.[39,43,63,69–80] Some have reported improvement when the breathing disorder was corrected.[43,63,71,73,74] Most of these studies were seriously flawed by small sample sizes, lack of control groups, or selection from special populations. These studies do suggest that SDB along with sleep disturbance may be associated with both cognitive and behavioral difficulties.

Enuresis is said to be a common feature of SDB,[44,81,82] but much of the data is based on anecdotal reports and uncontrolled case studies. Thus, the role of SDB as a cause for enuresis is unclear. Adenotonsillectomy often is the initial therapy for childhood SDB,[83–89] and SDB currently is one of the most common indications for adenotonsillectomy. Although SDB improves following surgery, the surgery includes a risk of intraoperative or postoperative death, hemorrhage, pain, airway compromise, and respiratory distress.[29] Finally, the likelihood of postoperative complications is greater for persons who have more severe SDB, younger age, less than optimal growth, and cardiovascular abnormalities.[83–86,88] Thus, a clear understanding of the clinical significance of all forms of SDB is important.

To date, several studies have evaluated the prevalence of SDB using objective sleep evaluation methods in general, random samples of children.[35–37,39–42] Five of these studies estimated the prevalence to be between 1% and 3%. One study reported the prevalence to be 12.0%, but this estimate was for "pathologic snoring." Another study did not report an estimated prevalence[42] but reported only that the incidence of apnea decreases with age in children aged 2 to 27 weeks. Five of these studies evaluated an children younger than 6 years,[35–37,41,42] and the other two evaluated children aged 2 to 18 years[39] and 8 to 11 years, respectively.[40] Two of these studies[36,37] used extremely small samples in their sleep laboratory phase (n = 11 and 10, respectively). Two other studies[35,39] used larger but still relatively small sample sizes of their laboratory phase "normal controls" (n = 132 and 126, respectively). None of these studies assessed the contribution of ear, nose, and throat abnormalities, and only one assessed the contribution of pulmonary abnormalities.[39] None of these studies used electrophysiologic measures to evaluate sleep; all relied only on indirect assessment. None of these studies evaluated general development (eg, height, weight, or age-adjusted body mass index [BMI]) as a possible outcome measure. None of these studies evaluated associations with clinical measures (eg, blood pressure). Only one study reported an association with daytime sleepiness.[35] This study also assessed behavior using the Connor Behavior Rating scale. No study evaluated academic progress.

APPLICATION OF HEART RATE VARIABILITY ANALYSIS TO ASSESS CARDIAC AUTONOMIC MODULATION

Analysis of beat-to-beat HRV, quantifying the variations of normal electrocardiography (ECG) R wave to R wave (RR) intervals, has emerged as a clinically and epidemiologically useful noninvasive method to assess cardiac autonomic activity quantitatively.[5–21] Most frequently, beat-to-beat RR interval data are collected from a Holter ECG recording or from a real-time ECG acquisition using a computer card attached to a computer with designated software algorithms. The Holter system allows regular mobility and activity and thus can be used to collect RR interval data over a prolonged period, but some Holter systems may have limited sampling frequency (about 200 Hz). The computerized ECG data acquisition system has sufficient sampling frequency and can be standardized to study protocols but limits participants' mobility (participants must remain in one position during the entire data acquisition period) and thus often is used for data acquisition over short periods (eg, 5–10 minutes). One requirement for RR interval collection is the sampling frequency. The optimal range is 250 to 500 Hz or higher.[21] When the sampling frequency is below 200 to 250 Hz, it may produce a jitter (an inaccuracy of 1–3 milliseconds) in the R wave fiducial point, thus leading to misclassification of RR intervals. Similarly, with a limited sampling rate, measurement errors in the high frequency components can increase as band frequency increases. The problems caused by a lower sampling frequency are especially important when short-term records are collected. Based on the authors' previous experience[20,22,24,90–100] and current recommendations,[21] however, even a 100-Hz sampling rate can be sufficient if appropriate sampling and interpolations are used in the HRV analysis, especially when analyzing long-term recordings.[101] Details of other technical requirements and recommendations have been published.[21]

In general, HRV analysis can produce the time and frequency domain HRV indices summarized in **Table 1**.

Previous work[5–24,90–100] has shown that heart rate oscillations at low frequencies (LF; ie, 0.04–0.15 Hz) are under the influence of both the sympathetic and parasympathetic nervous systems, whereas oscillations at high frequencies (HF; ie, 0.15–0.40 Hz) are under the influence of cardiac parasympathetic modulation only and have been used as a marker of parasympathetic activity. The LF/HF ratio has been used to represent the balance of sympathetic and parasympathetic control of the heart. Simple statistics from the analysis of beat-to-beat RR interval data are called "time domain HRV indices." The most frequently used time domain HRV indices include the standard deviation of all normal RR intervals (SDNN) and the square root of the mean squared differences of successive normal RR intervals (RMSSD). The SDNN corresponds closely to the total power of frequency domain analysis, and the RMSSD corresponds to HF from the frequency domain analysis.[21]

Studies of patient populations have found that lower HRV is associated with a higher risk of all-cause mortality and sudden cardiac death in survivors of acute myocardial infarction.[8–12] Results from population-based follow-up studies also suggest that impaired cardiac autonomic modulation measured by HRV is associated with the incidence of coronary heart disease, insulin resistance, hypertension, diabetes, the cluster of interrelated metabolic risk factors (metabolic syndrome), and various cardiac disease risk factors.[20,23,24,90–100] It has been proposed that HRV be used as a marker of cardiac vulnerability to arrhythmia and acute cardiac events.[21] Furthermore, evidence suggests that impaired heart rate variability may play a key role both as one of the consequences of central obesity, metabolic syndrome, sleep disorder, diabetes, and hypertension and also as the potential pathway between these conditions and the risk of clinical cardiac events.

It is well known that an episode of apnea is accompanied by a typical pattern of heart rate fluctuations (ie, bradycardia during the apneic phase and tachycardia at the restoration of ventilation). Several studies in adults have shown an association between SDB and lower HRV, indicating impaired cardiac autonomic modulation among persons who have SDB.[1–4] Sleep stages, even among persons who did not have SDB, were found to be associated with HRV: parasympathetic activity is highest in deep sleep and decreasing progressively in light sleep, rapid-eye movement (REM) sleep, and wakefulness; conversely, the heart rate is lower in deep sleep than in light sleep, lower in light sleep than in REM sleep, and lower in REM sleep than in a state of wakefulness. More importantly, this pattern of fluctuation in sympathetic and parasympathetic modulation was reduced in persons who had sleep apnea,[4] equivalent to diminished or reduced HRV circadian pattern. Recently data were presented[102] on the relationship of SDB and habitual snoring with lower HRV and prolonged QT intervals, indicative of the impaired cardiac autonomic modulation toward parasympathetic impairment and sympathetic overactivation among persons with SDB and habitual snoring.[103]

Table 1
Major heart rate variability (HRV) indices and their definitions

HRV Indices	Definition
SDNN	Standard deviation of all normal RR intervals (ms)
Mean HR	Mean heart rate (in beats per minute)
RMSSD	Square root of the mean of the sum of the squares of differences between adjacent normal RR intervals (in milliseconds)
SDANN	Standard deviation of the average of normal RR interval in all 5-minute segments of the entire long-term recording
SDANN Index	Mean of the standard deviations of all normal RR intervals for all 5-minute segments of the entire long-term recording
NN50	Number of pairs adjacent normal RR intervals differing by more than 50 milliseconds in the entire recording
pNN50	NN50 count divided by the total number of all normal RR interval (%)
RR_tri-index	Total number of all normal RR intervals divided by the height of the histogram of all normal RR intervals measured on a discrete scale with bins of 7.8125 milliseconds (1/128 seconds)
TiNN	Baseline width of the minimum square difference triangular interpolation the highest of the histogram of all normal RR intervals (in milliseconds)
VLF	Power in the very low frequency range (0.00–0.04 Hz)
LF	Power in the low frequency range (0.04–0.15 Hz)
HF	Power in the high frequency range (0.15–0.40 Hz)
LF/HF	Ratio of low frequency to high frequency
HF_nu	Normalized HF [HF/(LF + HF)] (expressed as a percentage)
LF_nu	Normalized LF [LF/(LF + HF)] (expressed as a percentage)

PRELIMINARY FINDINGS OF A POPULATION-BASED STUDY OF SLEEP-DISORDERED BREATHING, OBESITY, AND CARDIAC AUTONOMIC MODULATION

The authors have completed an NIH R01 grant titled "Prevalence of Sleep-Disordered Breathing in Children" (R01 HL063772) to recruit a population-based sample of young children and to investigate the prevalence of SDB and clinical correlates of SDB in this population. They also were awarded a R21 grant designed to retrieve and process the ECG data and to calculate frequency and time domain HRV variables as measures of cardiac autonomic modulation in the same population-based sample of young children (R21 HL087858: "Sleep-disordered Breathing, Sleep Stages and Heart Rate Variability in Children"). This section presents some of their preliminary findings using the HRV data generated from the R21 award to investigate cross-sectionally whether (1) SDB is associated with impaired cardiac autonomic modulation in young children; (2) whether sleep stage–specific cardiac modulation is altered in young children who have different degrees of SDB, and (3) whether cardiometabolic factors are associated impaired cardiac autonomic modulation in young children.

Population

The study population was from the Penn State Child Cohort (PSCC). The PSCC is a population-based study of the prevalence and correlates of SDB in children. Seven hundred children were enrolled in the baseline examination; the overall response rate was 70%. The mean age of participants was 9 years (SD ± 1.8 years); 48% of the participants were male, and 24% were nonwhite.

Methods

During the baseline examination, a detailed physical examination and a 9-hour standardized polysomnogram (PSG) recording were performed in the authors' sleep laboratory. The physical examination, completed during the evening before the PSG recording, included measurements of height, weight, and hip, waist, and neck circumferences, blood pressure, and pulmonary function. All measurements were based on standardized procedures and protocols and were subject to established quality control procedures.

From the 9-hour PSG in this population, a single-channel ECG was recorded continuously as voltages at a sampling rate of 100 Hz. The ECG data were retrieved, and the voltages were converted into waveforms. Then the peak of each QRS complex was identified as the R wave point, and beat-to-beat RR intervals for the entire night of ECG recording were calculated. An algorithm was applied to the entire RR interval data that identified and removed as artifacts any RR interval shorter than 375 milliseconds, any RR interval longer than 1200 milliseconds, or an RR interval ratio from two adjacent RR intervals less than 0.8 or greater than 1.2. Finally, HRV analysis was applied to the artifact-free RR interval files if the total length of the artifact-free RR interval file was more than 6.5 hours (corresponding to approximately 75% of the total recording time). The authors have calculated HRV data for 616 of the 700 participants (88%). From the HRV analysis, the HRV indices listed in **Table 1** were calculated. In addition to the HRV indices calculated from entire night (long-term) ECG data, sleep stage–specific short-term HRV indices were calculated based on the first available 5-minute continuous RR from each sleep stage.

The authors defined sleep apnea and hypopnea using criteria that are used currently in clinical practice.[104,105] All records were double scored. An apnea episode was defined as a cessation of airflow with a minimum duration of 5 seconds and an out-of-phase strain gauge movement. A hypopnea episode was defined as a reduction of airflow of approximately 50% with an associated decrease in oxygen saturation of at least 3% or an associated arousal. The total number of apnea and hypopnea episodes were combined and divided by the total duration of sleep to form the Apnea Hypopnea Index (AHI, episodes/hour of sleep). Individuals were identified as "without SDB" if the AHI was less than 1, as having "mild SDB" if the AHI was 1 or higher but less than 5, and as having "moderate SDB" if AHI was 5 or higher. In this population-based sample of young, healthy children, the average the AHI was 0.79 (SD 1.03); 73.8% had an AHI less than 1 (no SDB), 25.0% had an AHI between 1 and 5 (mild SDB), and 1.2% had an AHI of 5 or higher 5 (moderate SDB).

Major Preliminary Findings

Association of sleep-disordered breathing and long-term heart rate variability
The objective of this investigation was to investigate systematically the adverse cardiac autonomic effects of SDB in children.[25] After adjustments were made for age, race, sex, BMI, percentage of REM sleep, snore status, and sleep efficiency, children who had moderate SDB had significantly impaired cardiac autonomic modulation (as measured by both frequency and time domain HRV indices) than children who did not have SDB or children who had mild SDB. For example, among individuals who had moderate SDB, the mean of HRV-HF was significantly lower than in children without SDB, 6.00 (SE 0.32) versus 6.68 (SE 0.04) milliseconds squared ($P < .05$), whereas the LF/HF ratio was significantly higher, 1.62 (SE 0.20) versus 0.99 (SE 0.02) ($P < .01$). The authors concluded that, in this population-based sample of healthy young children, moderate SDB is associated significantly with impaired cardiac autonomic modulation (ie, sympathetic overflow unopposed by parasympathetic modulation). This association may contribute to the increased risk of acute cardiac events in persons who have SDB, even before they reach the traditional "high-risk" age,[106] but confirmation by further studies is needed.

Sleep-disordered breathing and impairment of sleep stage–specific shift of cardiac autonomic modulation in children
The objective of this study was to investigate the pattern of shifting of cardiac autonomic modulation across sleep stages (wakefulness, non-REM sleep, and REM sleep) in a population-based sample of young children and to investigate whether SDB has an adverse effect on the shifting of cardiac autonomic modulation in children.[107] The authors' sleep stage–specific 5-minute HRV data were used in this study. The data suggest that among children who do not have SDB, there is a significant increase in HRV indices and decrease in the LF/HF ratio from the wakeful stage to stage 2 sleep and slow-wavesleep, followed by a dramatic decrease in HRV indices and an increase in the LF/HF ratio when shifting into REM sleep. The multivariable adjusted means of log-HF were 5.80 (SE 0.05), 6.03 (SE 0.05), 6.02 (SE 0.05), and 5.39 (SE 0.05) milliseconds squared, for the wakefulness, stage 2 sleep, slow-wave sleep, and REM sleep, respectively, whereas the adjusted means of LF/HF ratio were 1.28 (SE 0.04), 0.91 (SE 0.04), 0.53 (SE 0.03), and 1.42 (SE 0.07), respectively, across the same sleep stages. Among children who had moderate SDB, the corresponding increases of HRV indices and decreases of LF/HF ratio from wakefulness to stage 2 sleep and slow-wave sleep were much less pronounced, whereas the corresponding decrease of HRV indices and the increase of LF/HF ratio from non-REM sleep to REM sleep was more

pronounced. The authors concluded that among healthy children there is a significant shift of the sympathetic and parasympathetic modulation of heart rhythm in the direction of reduced sympathetic outflow and increased parasympathetic modulation from wakefulness to non-REM sleep, and there is a significant reversal to sympathetic overflow and reduced parasympathetic modulation during REM sleep. Most importantly, this sympathetic–parasympathetic modulation shift across sleep stages is impaired in children who have moderate SDB, and this impairment may lead to increased vulnerability to arrhythmia during both REM and non-REM sleep.[107]

Association of sleep-disordered breathing and blood pressure is synergistically modified by lower heart rate variability

The authors have reported a significant association between SDB and blood pressure, especially systolic blood pressure, in this population-based cohort.[25] They performed additional analysis in this study to investigate whether the association between SDB and blood pressure can be explained by impaired cardiac autonomic modulation and whether there is a synergistic interaction between SDB and cardiac autonomic modulation in relation to blood pressure. They found that after adjustments for age, sex, race, BMI, REM sleep, sleep efficiency, and snoring, SDB was associated significantly with both blood pressure and HRV. Systolic blood pressure was 1.78 mm Hg higher in the mild SDB group and was 16.28 mm Hg higher in the moderate SDB group than in the no-SDB group. After additional adjustment of HRV indices, the difference in systolic blood pressure between the non-SDB group and the mild- and moderate SDB groups was reduced to 1.69 and 15.67 mm Hg, respectively, indicating that very little of the association between SDB and systolic blood pressure can be explained by HRV. The interactions between AHI and HRV indices in relation to systolic blood pressure were significant ($P < .05$): a higher AHI was associated with higher SBP at all levels of HRV indices, but the association was more pronounced among persons who had impaired HRV profiles. The authors concluded that in children the relationship between SDB and blood pressure is not mediated through the effects of SDB on cardiac autonomic modulation. Impaired cardiac autonomic modulation greatly enhanced the effects of SDB on systolic blood pressure, however.

Association of obesity and heart rate variability

The objective of this study was to investigate the effects of childhood obesity on cardiac autonomic modulation. The authors defined obesity according to age- and sex-specific BMI percentiles: children in the 85th percentile or lower were categorized as having normal weight; those between the 85th to 95th percentiles were categorized as being overweight, and those in the 95th percentile or higher were categorized as being obese. The overall prevalence of obesity was 15% (12.6%, 9.25%, 27.6%, and 27.6% for white boys, white girls, nonwhite boys, and nonwhite girls, respectively). After adjusting for age, sex, and race, the authors found a graded decline of HRV indices as weight increased from normal to obese. For example, the mean of log-transformed HF power was 6.82 (SE 0.04), 6.57 (SE 0.09), and 6.41 (SE 0.08) milliseconds squared, in the normal, overweight, and obese groups, respectively. Using linear regression analysis treating BMI, weight, and height percentiles as continuous variables, the authors also found that that the associations were strongest for HRV indices and weight percentile. They concluded that in this population-based sample of young children, obesity is associated significantly with impairment of cardiac autonomic modulation (ie, sympathetic overflow unopposed by parasympathetic modulation). These data support the need to target childhood obesity, even before children reach the "high-risk" age for acute cardiac events.

SUMMARY

Standardized beat-to-beat RR interval data can be collected for HRV analysis. The HRV indices in both the frequency and time domains have been used as noninvasive measures of cardiac autonomic modulation. In the cardiac disease literature, analysis of beat-to-beat HRV has emerged as a clinically and epidemiologically useful noninvasive method to assess cardiac autonomic activity quantitatively. Most importantly, lower HRV has been associated consistently with the risk of incident cardiovascular disease. HRV indices are used increasingly by researchers in the field of sleep medicine, but few studies in children have used HRV to assess cardiac autonomic modulation. In their population-based cohort of children, the authors observed significant cross-sectional associations between (1) impaired cardiac autonomic modulation and SDB; (2) impaired sleep stage specific cardiac autonomic modulation shift and SDB; (3) impaired cardiac autonomic modulation enhances the SDB effects on blood pressure; and (4) cardiac autonomic modulation impairment and obesity, independent of SDB. Therefore, it can be hypothesized that sleep-related disorders and childhood obesity can increase the risk of acute cardiac events even before the children reach the traditional "high-risk" age. These consistent findings also highlight the importance of a multidisciplinary approach extending research in sleep and sleep-related disorders into the field of cardiac disease. The lower HRV and the higher risk of acute cardiac events reported in the literature are based on studies in adults, and to date no data have been published regarding the association between childhood HRV and the future development of acute cardiac events. The authors' interpretation of the impact of SDB-related and obesity-related impairment of cardiac autonomic modulation in children is based on the premise of adult literature. Thus, further studies are required to determine whether lower HRV in children entails a higher risk of future acute cardiac events. Meanwhile, the authors' data also argue for more studies to evaluate the long-term effects of impaired cardiac autonomic modulation in childhood on cardiovascular disease.

REFERENCES

1. Guilleminault C, Connoly S, Winkle R, et al. Cyclical variation of heart rate in sleep apnoea syndrome. Lancet 1984;21:126–31.

2. Roche F, Pichot V, Sforza E, et al. Predicting sleep apnoea syndrome from heart rate period: a time-frequency wavelet analysis. Eur Respir J 2003;22: 937–42.

3. Clifford GD, Tarassenko L. Segmenting cardiac-related data using sleep stages increases separation between normal subjects and apnoeic patients. Physiol Meas 2004;25:N27–35.

4. Penzel T, Kantelhardt JW, Grote L, et al. Comparison of detrended fluctuation analysis and spectral analysis for heart rate variability in sleep apnea. IEEE Trans Biomed Eng 2003;50:1143–51.

5. Pfeifer MA, Cook D, Brodsky J, et al. Quantitative evaluation of cardiac parasympathetic activity in normal and diabetic man. Diabetes 1982;31: 339–45.

6. Bigger JT Jr. Spectral analysis of R-R variability to evaluate autonomic physiology and pharmacology and to predict cardiovascular outcomes in humans. In: Zipes D, Jalife J, editors. Cardiac electrophysiology: from the cell to the bedside. 2nd edition. Philadelphia: WB Saunders Co.; 1995. p. 1151–70.

7. Akselrod S, Gordon D, Ubel FA, et al. Power spectrum analysis of heart rate fluctuation: a quantitative probe of beat-to-beat cardiovascular control. Science 1981;213:220–2.

8. Pomeranz B, Macaulay RJ, Caudill MA, et al. Assessment of autonomic function in humans by heart rate spectral analysis. Am J Phys 1985;248: H151–3.

9. Hayano J, Sakakibara Y, Yamada A, et al. Accuracy of assessment of cardiac parasympathetic tone by heart rate variability in normal subjects. Am J Cardiol 1991;67:99–104.

10. Pagani M, Lombardi F, Guzzetti S, et al. Power spectral analysis of heart rate and arterial pressure variabilities as a marker of sympatho-parasympathetic interaction in man and conscious dog. Circ Res 1986;59:178–93.

11. Kamath MV, Ghista DN, Fallen EL, et al. Heart rate variability power spectrogram as a potential noninvasive signature of cardiac regulatory system response, mechanisms, and disorders. Heart Vessels 1987;3:33–41.

12. Malik M, Camm AJ. Heart rate variability. Clin Cardiol 1990;13:570–6.

13. Ori Z, Monir G, Weiss J, et al. Heart rate variability—frequency domain analysis. Cardiol Clin 1992;10:499–537.

14. Kleiger RE, Miller JP, Bigger JT Jr, et al. Decreased heart rate variability and its association with increased mortality after acute myocardial infarction. Am J Cardiol 1987;59:256–62.

15. Vaishnav S, Stevenson R, Marchant B, et al. Relation between heart rate variability early after acute myocardial infarction and long-term mortality. Am J Cardiol 1994;73:653–7.

16. Lombardi F, Sandrone G, Pernpruner S, et al. Heart rate variability as an index of sympathovagal interaction after acute myocardial infarction. Am J Cardiol 1987;60:1239–45.

17. Malik M, Farrell T, Camm AJ. Circadian rhythm of heart rate variability after acute myocardial infarction and its influence on the prognostic value of heart rate variability. Am J Cardiol 1990;66: 1049–54.

18. Martin GJ, Magid NM, Myers G, et al. Heart rate variability and sudden death secondary to coronary artery disease during ambulatory electrocardiographic monitoring. Am J Cardiol 1987;60: 86–9.

19. Tsuji H, Larson MG, Venditti FJ Jr, et al. Impact of reduced heart rate variability on cardiac events, The Framingham Heart Study. Circulation 1996; 94:2850–5.

20. Liao D, Cai J, Rosamond W, et al. Cardiac autonomic function and incident CHD: a population based case-cohort study—the ARIC study. Am J Epidemiol 1997;145:696–706.

21. Task Force of the European Society of Cardiology and the North American Society of Pacing and Electrophysiology: heart rate variability—standards of measurement, physiological interpretation, and clinical use. Circulation 1996;93:1043–65.

22. Dekker JM, Crow RS, Folsom AR, et al. Low heart rate variability in a two minute rhythm strip predicts risk of coronary heart disease and mortality from

several causes—the ARIC study. Circulation 2000; 102:1239–44.

23. Liao D, Carnethon MR, Evans GW, et al. Lower heart rate variability is associated with the development of coronary heart disease in individuals with diabetes—the ARIC study. Diabetes 2002;51: 3524–31.

24. Liao D, Cai Jianwen, Barnes RW, et al. Cardiac autonomic function and the development of hypertension—the ARIC study. Am J Hypertens 1996;9: 1147–56.

25. Bixler EO, Vgontzas AN, Lin H, et al. Blood pressure associated with sleep-disordered breathing in a population sample of children. Hypertension 2008;52:841–6.

26. Arens R. Obstructive sleep apnea in childhood: clinical features. In: Loughlin GM, Carroll JL, Marcus CL, editors. Sleep and breathing in children. New York: Marcel Dekker; 2000. p. 575–600.

27. Gaultier C. Obstructive sleep apnoea syndrome in infants and children: established facts and unsettled issues. Thorax 1995;50:1204–10.

28. Boudewyns AN, Van de Heyning PH. Obstructive sleep apnea syndrome in children: an overview. Acta Otorhinolaryngol Belg 1995;49:275–9.

29. Greene MG, Carroll JL. Consequences of sleep-disordered breathing in childhood. Curr Opin Pulm Med 1997;3:456–63.

30. Marcus CL. Pathophysiology of OSAS in children. In: Loughlin GM, Carroll JL, Marcus CL, editors. Sleep and breathing in children. New York: Marcel Dekker; 2000. p. 601–24.

31. Marcus CL. Clinical and pathophysiological aspects of obstructive sleep apnea in children. Pediatr Pulmonol Suppl 1997;16:123–4.

32. Brouillette R, Hanson D, David R, et al. A diagnostic approach to suspected obstructive sleep apnea in children. J Pediatr 1984;105:10–4.

33. Corbo GM, Cuciarelli F, Forest A, et al. Snoring in children: association with respiratory symptoms and passive smoke. BMJ 1989;71:74–6.

34. Teculescu DB, Caillier I, Perrin P, et al. Snoring in French preschool children. Pediatr Pulmonol 1992;13:239–44.

35. Ali NJ, Pitson DJ, Stradling JR. Snoring, sleep disturbance, and behaviour in 4–5 year olds. Arch Dis Child 1993;68:360–6.

36. Gislason T, Benediktsdottir B. Snoring, apneic episodes, and nocturnal hypoxemia among children 6 months to 6 years old: an epidemiologic study of lower limit of prevalence. Chest 1995; 107:963–6.

37. Hultcrantz E, Löfstrand-Tideström B, Ahlquist-Rastad J. The epidemiology of sleep related breathing disorder in children. Int J Pediatr Otorhinolaryngol 1995;32:S63–6.

38. Owen GO, Cantner RJ, Robinson A. Snoring, apnoea and ENT symptoms in the paediatric community. Clin Otolaryngol 1996;21:130–4.

39. Redline S, Tishler PV, Schluchter M, et al. Risk factors with obesity, race, and respiratory problems. Am J Respir Crit Care Med 1999;159: 1527–32.

40. Rosen CL, Larkin EL, Kirchner HL, et al. Prevalence and risk factors for sleep-disordered breathing in 8-to 11-year-old children: association with race and prematurity. J Pediatr 2003;142:383–9.

41. Castronovo V, Zucconi M, Nosetti L, et al. Prevalence of habitual snoring and sleep-disordered breathing in preschool-aged children in an Italian community. J Pediatr 2003;142:377–82.

42. Kato I, Franco P, Groswasser J, et al. Frequency of obstructive and mixed sleep apneas in 1,023 infants. Sleep 2000;23:487–92.

43. Brouillette RT, Fernbach SK, Hunt CE. Obstructive sleep apnea in infants and children. J Pediatr 1982;100:31–40.

44. Guilleminault C, Korobkin R, Winkle R. A review of 50 children with obstructive sleep apnea syndrome. Lung 1981;159:275–87.

45. Redline S, Tishler PV, Hans MG, et al. Racial differences in sleep-disordered breathing in African-Americans and Caucasians. Am J Respir Crit Care Med 1997;155:186–92.

46. Goodwin JL, Babar SI, Kaemingk KI, et al. Symptoms related to sleep-disordered breathing in white and Hispanic children. Chest 2003;124: 196–203.

47. Redline S, Tishler PV, Tosteson TD, et al. The familial aggregation of obstructive sleep apnea. Am J Respir Crit Care Med 1995;151:682–7.

48. Redline S, Tosteson T, Tishler PV, et al. Studies in the genetics of obstructive sleep apnea: familial aggregation of symptoms associated with sleep-related breathing disturbances. Am Rev Respir Dis 1992;145:440–4.

49. Marcus CL, Crockett DM, Davidson-Ward SL. Evaluation of epiglottoplasty as treatment for severe laryngomalacia. J Pediatr 1990;117:706–10.

50. Kaihn A, Grosswasser J, Sottiaux M, et al. Prenatal exposure to cigarettes in infants with obstructive sleep apneas. Pediatrics 1994;93:778–83.

51. Grundfast KM, Wittich DJ Jr. Adenotonsillar hypertrophy and upper airway obstruction in evolutionary perspective. Laryngoscope 1982;92:650–6.

52. Mangat D, Orr WC, Smith RO. Sleep apnea, hypersomnolence, and upper airway obstruction secondary to adenotonsillar enlargement. Arch Otolaryngol 1977;103:383–6.

53. Goldstein NA, Post JC, Rosenfeld RM, et al. Impact of tonsillectomy and adenoidectomy on child behavior. Arch Otolaryngol Head Neck Surg 2000;126:494–8.

54. Sofer S, Weinhouse E, Tal A, et al. Cor pulmonale due to adenoidal or tonsillar hypertrophy or both in young children: noninvasive diagnosis and follow-up. Chest 1988;93:119–22.

55. Levy AM, Tabakin BS, Hanson JS, et al. Hypertrophied adenoids causing pulmonary hypertension and severe congestive heart failure. N Engl J Med 1967;397:506–11.

56. Hunt CE, Brouillette RT. Abnormalities of breathing control and airway maintenance in infants and children as a cause of cor pulmonale. Pediatr Cardiol 1982;3:249–56.

57. Levine OR, Simpson M. Alveolar hypoventilation and cor pulmonale associated with chronic airway obstruction in infants with Down syndrome. Clin Pediatr (Phila) 1982;21:25–9.

58. Serratto M, Harris VJ, Carr I. Upper airways obstruction: presentation with systemic hypertension. Arch Dis Child 1981;56:153–5.

59. Enright PI, Goodwin JL, Sherrill DL, et al. Blood pressure elevation associated with sleep-related breathing disorder in a community sample of white and Hispanic children. Arch Pediatr Adolesc Med 2003;157:901–4.

60. Guilleminault C, Eldridge FL, Simmons FB, et al. Sleep apnea in eight children. Pediatrics 1976;58:23–30.

61. Butt W, Robertson C, Phelan P. Snoring in children: is it pathological? Med J Aust 1985;143:335–6.

62. Praud JP, DAllest AM, Nedelcoux H, et al. Sleep-related abdominal muscle behavior during partial or complete obstructed breathing in prepubertal children. Pediatr Res 1989;26:347–50.

63. Guilleminault C, Winkle R, Korobkin R, et al. Children and nocturnal snoring: evaluation of the effects of sleep related respiratory resistive load and daytime functioning. Eur J Pediatr 1982;139:165–71.

64. Lind MG, Lundell BP. Tonsillar hyperplasia in children: a cause of obstructive sleep apneas, CO_2 retention, and retarded growth. Arch Otolaryngol 1982;108:650–4.

65. Stradling JR, Thomas G, Warley AR, et al. Effect of adenotonsillectomy on nocturnal hypoxaemia, sleep disturbance, and symptoms in snoring children. Lancet 1990;335:249–53.

66. Freezer NJ, Bucens IK, Robertson CF. Obstructive sleep apnoea presenting as failure to thrive in infancy. J Paediatr Child Health 1995;1:172–5.

67. Marcus CL, Koerner CB, Carroll JL, et al. Determinants of growth failure in children with obstructive sleep apnea syndrome. J Pediatr 1994;125:556–62.

68. Goldstein SJ, Wu RH, Thorpy MJ, et al. Reversibility of deficient sleep entrained growth hormone secretion in a boy with achondroplasia and obstructive sleep apnea. Acta Endocrinol (Copenh) 1987;116:95–101.

69. Weissbluth M, David AT, Poncher J, et al. Signs of airway obstruction during sleep and behavioral, developmental, and academic problems. J Dev Behav Pediatr 1983;4:119–21.

70. Rhodes SK, Shimoda KC, Waid LR, et al. Neurocognitive deficits in morbidly obese children with obstructive sleep apnea. J Pediatr 1995;127:741–4.

71. Martin PR, Lefebvre AM. Surgical treatment of sleep-apnea-associated psychosis. Can Med Assoc J 1981;124:978–80.

72. Ali NJ, Pitson D, Stradling JR. Sleep disordered breathing: effects of adenotonsillectomy on behaviour and psychological functioning. Eur J Pediatr 1996;155:56–62.

73. Lopez-Herce Cid J, Garcia Teresa MA, Ruiz Beltran A, et al. Obstructive sleep apnea syndrome in childhood: study of three cases. An Esp Pediatr 1991;35:347–9.

74. Kaemingk KL, Pasvogel AE, Goodwin JL, et al. Learning in children and sleep disordered breathing: findings of the Tucson Children's Assessment of Sleep Apnea (TuCASA) prospective cohort study. J Int Neuropsychol Soc 2003;9:1016–26.

75. Golan N, Shahar E, Ravid S, et al. Sleep disorders and daytime sleepiness in children with attention-deficit/hyperactive disorder. Sleep 2004;27:261–6.

76. Gruber R, Sadeh A. Sleep and neurobehavioral functioning in boys with attention-deficit/hyperactivity disorder and no reported breathing problems. Sleep 2004;27:267–73.

77. O'Brien LM, Tauman R, Gozal D. Sleep pressure correlates of cognitive and behavioral morbidity in snoring children. Sleep 2004;27:279–82.

78. Chervin RD, Archbold KH. Hyperactivity and polysomnographic findings in children evaluated for sleep-disordered breathing. Sleep 2001;24:313–20.

79. Gozal D. Sleep-disordered breathing and school performance in children. Pediatrics 1998;102:616–20.

80. Gozal D, Pope DW. Snoring during early childhood and academic performance at ages thirteen to fourteen years. Pediatrics 2001;107:1394–9.

81. Frank Y, Kravath RE, Pollak CP, et al. Obstructive sleep apnea and its therapy: clinical and polysomnographic manifestations. Pediatrics 1983;71:737–42.

82. Guilleminault C, Stoohs R. Obstructive sleep apnea syndrome in children. Pediatrician 1990;17:46–51.

83. Gerber ME, ÓConnor DM, Adler E, et al. Selected risk factors in pediatric adenotonsillectomy. Arch Otolaryngol Head Neck Surg 1996;122:811–4.

84. McColley SA, April MM, Carroll JL, et al. Respiratory compromise after adenotonsillectomy in children with obstructive sleep apnea. Arch Otolaryngol Head Neck Surg 1992;118:940–3.

85. Rosen GM, Muckle RP, Mahowald MW, et al. Postoperative respiratory compromise in children with obstructive sleep apnea syndrome: can it be anticipated? Pediatrics 1994;93:784–8.

86. Price SD, Hawkins DB, Kahlstrom EJ. Tonsil and adenoid surgery for airway obstruction: perioperative respiratory morbidity. Ear Nose Throat J 1993; 72:526–31.

87. Wiatrak BJ, Myer CM III, Andrews TM. Complications of adenotonsillectomy in children under 3 years of age. Am J Otol 1991;12:170–2.

88. Rothschild MA, Catalano P, Biller HF. Ambulatory pediatric tonsillectomy and the identification of high-risk subgroups. Otolaryngol Head Neck Surg 1994;110:203–10.

89. Williams EF III, Woo P, Miller R, et al. The effects of adenotonsillectomy on growth in young children. Otolaryngol Head Neck Surg 1991;104: 509–16.

90. Liao D, Barnes RW, Chambless LE, et al. Population based study of heart rate variability and prevalent myocardial infraction—the ARIC study. J Electrocardiol 1996;29:189–98.

91. Liao D, Creason J, Shy C, et al. Daily variation of particulate air pollution and poor cardiac autonomic control in the elderly. Environ Health Perspect 1999;107:521–5.

92. Liao D, Sloan RP, Cascio WE, et al. The multiple metabolic syndrome is associated with lower heart rate variability—the ARIC study. Diabetes Care 1998;21:2116–22.

93. Carnethon MR, Liao D, Evans GW, et al. Does the cardiac autonomic response to postural change predict incident coronary heart disease and mortality? The Atherosclerosis Risk in Communities study. Am J Epidemiol 2002;155:48–56.

94. Carnethon MR, Liao D, Evans GW, et al. Correlates of the shift in heart rate variability with an active postural change in a healthy population sample: the Atherosclerosis Risk In Communities study. Am Heart J 2002;143:808–13.

95. Carnethon MR, Golden SH, Folson AR, et al. Prospective association between hormone replacement therapy and heart rate variability: the Atherosclerosis Risk in Communities study. J Clin Epidemiol 2003;56:565–71.

96. Mercedes Carnethon R, Sherita Golden H, Aaron R. Folsom, et al. Prospective investigation of autonomic nervous system function and the development of type 2 diabetes: the Atherosclerosis Risk in Communities study, 1987–1998. Circulation 2003;107:2190–5.

97. Schroeder Emily B, Welch Verna Lamar, Couper David, et al. Lung function and incident coronary heart disease—the Atherosclerosis Risk in Communities study. Am J Epidemiol 2003;158:1171–81.

98. Emily Schroeder B, Liao Duanping, Chambless Lloyd E, et al. Hypertension, blood pressure, and heart rate variability: the Atherosclerosis Risk in Communities (ARIC) study. Hypertension 2003;42:1106–11.

99. Liao Duanping, Duan Yinkang, Whitsel EA, et al. Higher ambient criteria pollutants are associated with impaired cardiac autonomic control—a population-based study. Am J Epidemiol 2004;159: 768–77.

100. Schroeder EB, Chambless LE, Liao D, et al. Diabetes, glucose, insulin, and heart rate variability: the Atherosclerosis Risk in Communities (ARIC) study. Diabetes Care 2005;28:668–74.

101. Bianchi AM, Mainardi LT, Petrucci E, et al. Time-variant power spectrum analysis for the detection of transient episodes in HRV signal. IEEE Trans Biomed Eng 1993;40:136–44.

102. Javier-Nieto F, Peppard P, Szklo-Coxe M, et al. Sleep apnea, insulin resistance, and endothelial function in the Wisconsin sleep cohort. Abstracts of 46th AHA Council on CVD Epidemiology meeting Phoenix, AZ, March 2–5, 2006.

103. Kim E, Choi H, Kim J, et al. Association of QT interval with habitual snoring in middle aged population. Abstracts of 46th AHA Council on CVD Epidemiology meeting Phoenix, AZ, March 2–5, 2006.

104. Standards and indications for cardiopulmonary sleep studies in children. American Thoracic Society. Am J Respir Crit Care Med 1996;153: 866–78.

105. American Academy of Pediatrics. Clinical practice guidelines: diagnosis and management of childhood obstructive sleep apnea syndrome. Pediatrics 2002;109:704–12.

106. Liao D, Duan Y, Liu J, et al. Cardiac autonomic effects of sleep-disordered breathing in children: Penn State Child Cohort [abstract]. AHA 48th Annual Conference on Cardiovascular Disease Epidemiology. March 12–15. Colorado Springs, CO. Circulation 2008;117(28):E204 A.

107. Liao D, Duan D, Vgontzas AN, et al. Cardiac autonomic effects of sleep-disordered breathing in children: Penn State Child Cohort [abstract]. 22nd Annual Meeting of the Associated Professional Sleep Societies. June 7–12, 2008. Baltimore, MD. Sleep 2008;31:A143.0428.

Rationale, Design, and Findings from the Wisconsin Sleep Cohort Study: Toward Understanding the Total Societal Burden of Sleep-Disordered Breathing

Terry Young, PhD

KEYWORDS

- Obstructive sleep apnea • Sleep disorder
- Epidemiology • Public health • Cohort study

Over the past 2 decades, clinical and public health recognition of the importance of sleep-disordered breathing (SDB) and other sleep disorders has increased markedly.[1–5] Findings from epidemiology studies, many of which were presented at the University of Pennsylvania–Hershey symposium (November 2007, "Epidemiology of Sleep Disorders: Clinical Implications") have been critical in identifying the high prevalence of undiagnosed SDB and in linking this disorder with significant morbidity.[6–15] Identification of the high prevalence of undiagnosed SDB by population-based studies in the 1990s contributed to the growing increase in clinical recognition of SDB. The increase in clinical interest, in turn, prompted the need for additional epidemiology studies to quantify the adverse health outcomes of this condition, to determine the total societal burden of SDB. Thus, the rationale for the Wisconsin Sleep Cohort Study (WSCS) and other population-based studies, and the significance of findings, must be explained in the context of the fascinating history of sleep medicine.

This article is not a general review of SDB: The assignment for this article was to elaborate on the presentation at the Hershey Symposium. This report is a summary of research of the WSCS, not a review of the epidemiology of sleep apnea. Consequently, references are restricted to WSCS findings and studies that contributed to the design of the WSCS. Since then, many ongoing population-based studies have made important contributions that address the overall question of the burden of SDB but they are beyond the scope of this article and could not be included.

RATIONALE FOR A POPULATION-BASED COHORT STUDY OF SLEEP-DISORDERED BREATHING: 1960 TO 1987
The Emerging Need to Understand the Health Burden of Sleep-Disordered Breathing

In this article, SDB refers to the condition of repeated apnea and hypopnea events during sleep, most commonly indicated by the number of apnea and hypopnea events per hour of sleep

This work was supported by grants R01HL62252, RR03186, and R01AG14124 from the National Institutes of Health.

Department of Population Health Sciences, School of Medicine and Public Health, University of Wisconsin-Madison, 1070 SMC, 1300 University Avenue, Madison WI 53705, USA

E-mail address: tbyoung@wisc.edu

Sleep Med Clin 4 (2009) 37–46
doi:10.1016/j.jsmc.2008.11.003

(apnea-hypopnea index [AHI]). (Because most apnea and hypopnea events detected in population studies are due to upper airway collapse and increased airway resistance, with few events due to lack of respiratory muscle activation [central apnea], SDB is used in this report to reflect mainly obstructive sleep apnea.) This anomaly of breathing pauses during sleep was documented centuries ago by scholars using colorful case descriptions, usually combined with the common symptom of daytime sleepiness.[16,17] However, it was not until 1966 that European researchers and clinicians clearly defined the clinical entity of sleep apnea syndrome (SAS) as the combination of episodes of obstructive apnea and daytime symptoms, particularly extreme daytime sleepiness.[18] At that time, the only effective treatment of SDB was a tracheotomy to provide a patent surgical airway in the cervical trachea. With only an invasive treatment to offer, only the most severe cases of sleep apnea were likely to come to medical attention. Clinical interest in sleep apnea and other sleep disorders remained low in most countries, including the United States, with notable exceptions. In the United States, Stanford researchers, led by Drs. Dement and Guilleminault, persisted in forming a key research and clinical foundation devoted to sleep disorders, including SDB. With a small group of dedicated researchers, an early professional society was formed and the groundwork for a new field was set in place.[5]

During this critical time, in 1981, Sullivan[19] introduced a revolutionary new treatment of sleep apnea: continuous positive airway pressure (CPAP). CPAP, delivered by a small facial mask, effectively kept the upper airway patent and prevented episodes of SDB.

Of profound importance, a treatment of SDB that was acceptable to patients had become available and because it was now a feasibly treatable disorder, the significance of SDB greatly increased.

Dr. Dement's efforts to overcome the barriers to research and clinical care of sleep disorders were unrelenting, and by 1986 had reached the US Congress. The result was a task force and a congressional mandate to determine the state of knowledge of sleep disorders and resource needs and to seek a new National Institutes of Health commitment to research.[20] An important part of the charge to the task force was to determine the overall public burden of SDB. The Heart, Lung, and Blood Institute began to promote research in SDB with workshops to identify research needs, and then, in 1987, requested grant applications for specialized centers for cardiopulmonary disorders of sleep that would combine clinical, experimental, and epidemiologic research programs. As the epidemiologic component of the grant application from the University of Wisconsin, we proposed the WSCS, a longitudinal epidemiology study designed to investigate the natural history of SDB by conducting overnight polysomnography (PSG) studies on a random sample of the general population.

Motivation for Population-Based Studies to Determine the Total Societal Burden of Sleep-Disordered Breathing

To address the congressional mandate and identify long-term research goals, an accurate description of the public health burden of SDB was needed. As shown in **Fig. 1**, the health burden of a disorder is the product of the prevalence and the proportion of adverse health outcomes that can be attributed to the disorder. Two decades ago, virtually all information about SDB prevalence and outcomes was based on observations of the few patients, mostly men, diagnosed with SDB.[6,7] Although it was considered an uncommon disorder, clinical studies linked significant morbidity and mortality with SDB. Clinical researchers found excessive daytime sleepiness, motor vehicle crashes, hypertension, cardiovascular disease, and mortality to be more prevalent in patients who had SDB.[21,22] Thus, 2 decades ago, estimating the total health burden of SDB was limited by lack of a valid estimate of how many people were affected by this disorder. Furthermore, clinic referral and other biases and limitations in control groups raised concern that the health risks linked with SDB morbidity were overestimated. Although CPAP clearly reduced apnea and hypopnea episodes, outside of the small field of sleep research, the lack of rigorous trials of CPAP efficacy was criticized.

At the time the WSCS was designed, only a few people who had SDB had been diagnosed and treated. Compared with most medical specialties, established in the mid-1800s, sleep medicine was still in its early years: it was not until 1994 that sleep medicine was recognized by the American Medical Association as a subspecialty.

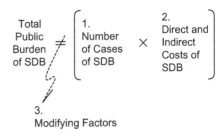

Fig. 1. The total public burden of SDB.

Consequently, general medical training and resources for recognition of SDB and other sleep disorders were rare. Although awareness of SDB has grown, the increase in case finding has not been uniform, either intra- or internationally.

The striking and unpredictable growth in clinical and public recognition of SDB presents a challenge for determining the occurrence of SDB and investigating SDB risk factors and adverse long-term health consequences. In common with other disorders with low and uneven recognition by the health care system, the patients who had SDB who were evaluated and diagnosed have been different in known and unknown ways from most cases of SDB that remain undetected. This phenomenon of selective referral and diagnosis for underrecognized but prevalent disorders is recognized in epidemiology as the "tip of the iceberg" paradigm, whereby the iceberg comprises all cases of SDB and multiple factors determine which cases ultimately become "patients" who have diagnosed SDB.

As shown in **Fig. 2**, many forces shape referral patterns for SDB, beginning with the individual seeking care. In the past, the symptoms of SDB, including snoring and daytime sleepiness, were not seen by the general public as indicators of a medical problem, but rather as comical characteristics or a nuisance, at best. Thus, individuals told they were loud snorers or always sleeping

were unlikely to seek care for SDB symptoms. Until recently, SDB was most likely to be diagnosed only incidentally, while a patient was being seen for a different medical complaint. A patient hospitalized for a myocardial infarct, for example, might be observed to stop breathing during sleep, and a consultation with a sleep specialist, if available, might be sought. Consequently, SDB was more likely to be diagnosed in someone who had comorbid conditions, which may or may not have been related to SDB. Further bias is introduced because access to any health care is limited by socioeconomic status, thereby confounding correlates of SDB with those of education and income. The view of the stereotypic patient who has SDB was that of an overweight, sleepy, middle-aged, snoring man, resulting in a referral bias against women and older patients. Even with optimal awareness in primary care, the ability to refer a patient is tempered by the perceived severity of SDB symptoms, availability of a sleep clinic, patient willingness, and ability to pay. These and other selection biases serve to build in spurious associations of SDB with other characteristics and disorders. Consequently, the characteristics of SDB patients are clinic specific, and using sleep clinic patient samples to address questions regarding risk factors, causes, and consequences of SDB may not be generalizable beyond the specific clinic sample. As a result,

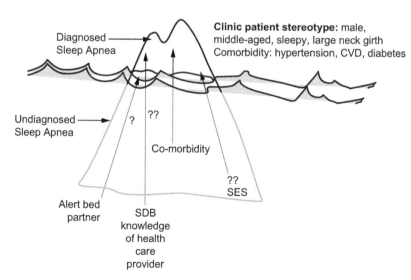

SELECTION FACTORS

Fig. 2. Selection biases for clinical recognition and diagnosis of sleep apnea. The proportion of all cases of sleep apnea is represented by the iceberg, with clinically diagnosed cases shown in the tip of the iceberg. Clinically recognized sleep apnea represents less than 85% of the total prevalence of sleep apnea cases that would be candidates for treatment. Factors that favor selection of individuals who have unrecognized sleep apnea (below the tip of the iceberg) for clinical referral and diagnosis are shown. CVD, cerebrovascular disease; SES, socioeconomic status.

epidemiology studies of SDB in population samples, free of clinic selection biases and designed to minimize other biases, were critical to determine the health burden of SDB and to provide a foundation for developing clinical and public health strategies.

DESIGN OF THE WISCONSIN SLEEP COHORT STUDY

The primary goal of the WSCS was to investigate the natural history of SDB and other sleep disorders, with the long-term goal of better understanding the total societal burden of SDB. Specifically, our aims were to (1) describe occurrence, including age- and sex-specific prevalence for mild, moderate, and severe SDB; (2) estimate, with longitudinal data, the role of SDB in cardiovascular and behavioral morbidity and mortality; and (3) identify risk factors for the development and progression of SDB. The fundamental components for the study design were those of a standard epidemiology prospective cohort study, including the identification of a population-based sampling frame, recruitment of a probability sample with sufficient variation in exposure and adequate power for hypothesis testing, and collection of data with sufficient accuracy at baseline and follow-up. A major factor influencing the WSCS design was the decision to use in-laboratory PSG for describing SDB. PSG was the clinical diagnostic standard for identifying SDB; thus, use of PSG in our population study would provide comparable findings that could be translated to the clinical setting. Furthermore, the extensive data recorded by PSG provide many parameters for measurement accuracy (ie, breathing by sleep stage), redundancy, and flexibility in operational definitions of breathing events. However, in-laboratory, standard PSG was expensive and labor intensive, and a participant burden. In previous studies, when PSG was the measurement tool of choice, sample sizes were generally smaller; large studies tended to use objective monitoring with fewer signals or subjective indicators of SDB, such as self-reported snoring.

Influence of Early Population-Based Studies

To help plan several aspects of the WSCS design, we relied on the few pioneering studies of SDB in the population published before 1988.[8,11–15] These studies provided the first impressions of the occurrence of undiagnosed SDB and revealed general and unique methodologic problems in quantifying SDB prevalence and in investigating associations of SDB with adverse health consequences.

Bliwise and colleagues[12] reported on the first population cohort of 198 middle-aged and older people screened for SDB by in-laboratory PSG and followed over time. In addition to finding a high prevalence, the investigators investigated night-to-night variability in SDB, thereby first bringing attention to the need for study designs to accommodate this measurement error. Bliwise and colleagues[13] also noted the high prevalence with age, the progression in the respiratory distress index (breathing events per hour of sleep) over a 10-year period, and the risk for cardiovascular death.[14] In Europe, in 1983, Lavie[11] reported findings from a two-stage approach to screen for SDB symptoms in Israeli industrial workers. The group was surveyed for SDB symptoms, with the expectation that almost all cases of SDB would be concentrated in the group reporting symptoms. PSG was then performed on the symptomatic sample to obtain a "minimum" prevalence. A prevalence of 1% resulted.

Using in-home monitoring without electroencephalogram, Ancoli-Israel and colleagues[15] screened sleep and breathing in a sample of 358 elderly community dwelling volunteers with a mean age of 72 years. Reported in 1987, the prevalence of obstructive sleep apnea was estimated at 31% in men and 19% in women. Central sleep apnea was found in 6% of the sample.

In 1987, Gislason and Taube[23] meticulously described the statistical considerations and methodologic concerns that shaped the design of an investigation of SDB prevalence in Swedish men. Limited by resources for in-laboratory monitoring, the researchers determined the enriched sampling scheme needed that would result in adequate variation in a subsample of 60 men symptomatic for SDB. Taking these calculations and participation rate into account, a postal survey was sent to 4064 men. Men who reported snoring sometimes or more often and daytime sleepiness formed the high-risk group; a total of 166 were identified from the survey responses and recruited for the overnight study. Taking a conservative approach that all SDB cases were captured in the high-risk category, results from the 60 participants were extrapolated to the sampling frame of 30- to 69-year-old men, concluding that the minimal prevalence of SDB was 1.3%.[8] Thus, at the time the WSCS was designed, the sparse information available suggested that SDB prevalence was markedly different in the United States and European populations, and differed by age. It was not clear if the wide variability in prevalence was due to participant characteristics including age and gender, sampling error, or differences in methods of quantifying SDB. Based on the previous studies, it was clear that to address our aims we needed a probability sampling scheme to yield a final cohort sample enriched for SDB risk of approximately 800 middle-aged men and women. We chose an age range of 30 to 60, with the expectation that we would be able to monitor SDB prevalence from middle to older age with overnight studies at baseline and at follow-up intervals of 4 years. Drawing on the methods of Gislason, we planned a two-stage sampling scheme to increase variability in SDB and thereby increase study power.[24]

Sample Construction

Identification of a sampling frame, or enumeration of individuals with a known chance of being sampled, was our first requirement. For this, we chose the payroll files of Wisconsin State employees in the year 1988. The sampling frame had several advantages. It comprised a complete range of jobs, from unskilled to professional, and included sociodemographic data on the entire sampling frame for targeted recruitment and for eventual comparison of responders and nonresponders. Like other employed groups, the sample could be traced more easily, an important advantage for longitudinal studies. Furthermore, cohorts based on defined employee groups often have a positive identity that increases commitment to the study. All employees had equal access to health care, an advantage in reducing potential bias in health outcomes. The payroll file data included contact information, social security number, details on job, pay rate, sex, birth date, race and other factors.

All employees aged 30 to 60 in 1988 and living or working in a defined area of south central Wisconsin were eligible for sample selection. Using a two-stage scheme, a mailed survey was sent to a random sample of the eligible sampling frame and a subsample was recruited from the respondents for the longitudinal cohort study. The survey included questions on sociodemographics, life style, health habits, and sleep characteristics. A variable for SDB high risk was based on answers to questions on snoring frequency and loudness, and breathing pauses. A survey respondent was considered to be high risk if he or she reported snoring sometimes or more frequently or very loud snoring, or had witnessed breathing pauses, and the remainder were considered low risk. We did not introduce sleepiness into the risk definition because this would hinder assessment of the independent role of SDB in daytime impairment. All high-risk respondents and an age- and sex-matched random sample of low-risk respondents

were recruited, with approximately 1.5:1.0 weighting of high/low risk. This technique is commonly used for increasing study power. The weighted sampling scheme is accounted for with specialized software.

After the cohort sample was constructed, the potential participants were recruited for the cohort overnight study protocol by repeated mailed invitations and by telephone, at a rate to perform eight in-laboratory studies per week. To meet our target enrollment, we anticipated baseline studies would be performed continuously for about 3 to 4 years, after which time we would begin 4-year follow-up studies. The sample design and baseline protocol are shown in **Fig. 3**. Over the next several years, other protocols were added and ancillary studies were conducted. We continued enrollment beyond the original target of 900, for a total of 1550 men and women. This sample continues to cycle through follow-up studies, in synchrony with the rolling recruitment over the first 3 years. As a result, the earliest participants have had the opportunity for five follow-up studies, whereas later participants are being recruited currently for their third study.

The defined sampling frame for the first stage sample allowed us to examine potential participation bias on sociodemographic factors and other data that could be linked, including mortality records. The survey respondents comprised the second-stage sampling frame, from which we recruited the cohort participants. The more detailed data from the survey on the entire sampling frame were vital in comparing nonparticipants, participants, and those who dropped out of the cohort.

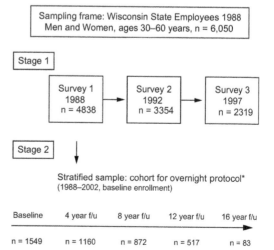

Fig. 3. Wisconsin Sleep Cohort Study design and protocol. A two-stage sampling design was used to obtain the WSCS sample for baseline and 4-year follow-up overnight protocols. The basic study protocol is listed.

The participation rate was 82% for the survey stage, and nonrespondents did not differ from respondents on the sociodemographic variables. Participation for the baseline overnight protocol rose from 50% to 54% by completion. Based on survey data, participants showed a typical healthy volunteer bias, with less self-reported hypertension and slightly higher education. Comparisons of participants and nonparticipants have been analysis specific (eg, stratified by gender, SDB findings, and many other factors).[24–26] In a study of SDB and mortality, we were able in explore possible retention bias by comparing the mortality of participants who withdrew from the longitudinal study.[26] Mortality was higher for survey participants who did not participate in the cohort, than for the participants. The elevated mortality rate was found for both risk groups of the nonparticipants (high and low SDB risk, based on survey data). Thus, a healthy volunteer bias, commonly seen in epidemiology cohort studies, has been consistent at all stages of the study. The "better health" bias did not differ by the important study factors of SDB, so it is unlikely that our findings overestimated the health risks of SDB. However, it is likely that having a slightly healthier cohort resulted in a loss of study power and the ability to detect small differences in outcomes by SDB status. In addition, it is possible that the prevalence of SDB was underestimated at the baseline.

FINDINGS FROM THE WISCONSIN SLEEP COHORT STUDY

In keeping with the original long-term goal of determining the total societal burden of SDB, the most relevant findings from the WSCS are described below, organized into the three components of the total burden: the number of affected people, the cost of SDB, and the effects of modifying factors.

The Number of People Affected with Sleep-Disordered Breathing: Prevalence by Age and Sex

Our estimates of prevalence required careful extrapolation to account for the two-stage sampling procedure to increase SDB variance (ie, oversampling habitual, loud snorers and those with reported breathing pauses).[24] As reported in 1993, with SDB severity indicated by the AHI, we found a wide severity spectrum, with AHI ranging from 0 to 92. Using commonly used cut points (AHI at 5 and 15) to indicate mild, moderate, and severe SDB, we estimated the age- and sex-specific prevalence as weighted averages from the high- and low-risk strata. The age- and

sex-specific prevalence estimates could then be applied to any other population with different age and sex distributions. The overall prevalence for AHI 5 to 15 and AHI greater than 15 based on the cohort distribution of age was also calculated, showing a markedly high prevalence for SDB for both men and women. Prevalence (95% confidence interval) of having SDB with an AHI greater than 5 was 9% (95% CI 5.6–12.0) for women and 24% for men, and for AHI greater than 15 was 4% (95% CI 1.5–6.6) for women and 9% (95% CI 6.4–11.0) for men. We also calculated prevalence of SDB with daytime sleepiness as a surrogate for clinically diagnosed sleep apnea syndrome. For this, we used a strict definition of sleepiness: Using three standard questions about sleepiness (falling asleep against wishes, not feeling rested regardless of hours of sleep, and sleepiness that affects daily functioning), participants were categorized as having excessive daytime sleepiness if they answered all three questions positively. The prevalence of SAS, based on AHI greater than 5 and "excessive daytime sleepiness" was 2% for women and 4% for men. It is important to note that the prevalence for SAS would have been higher if we had used a less stringent definition of excessive daytime sleepiness. Similarly, in our study, a 4% desaturation is required for a hypopnea event; prevalence would obviously be higher if our definition included events with a 3% desaturation. As other researchers have formally reported, prevalence of any disorder is highly dependent on definitions and cut points.

Describing the high prevalence and wide severity spectrum was an important step toward addressing the societal burden of SDB. Since our report, several other studies, using comparable methods, have reported similar SDB prevalence.[9,10,27] The high prevalence of screen-detected SDB, compared with the few patients diagnosed with SDB, indicated that a large proportion of people who have SDB who would meet clinical criteria for treatment were not being diagnosed. Furthermore, the findings revealed a gender bias: Although SDB was more prevalent than expected in general, this was particularly striking for women. In sleep clinic populations, the ratio of men to women who had SDB was approximately 9:1, but in the general population, at equal severity, the ratio was 2 to 3:1. This difference indicated a strong bias against women being diagnosed with SDB.[25]

SDB prevalence varies with population differences in the prevalence of SDB risk factors, including overweight/obesity (a strong causal factor) and age. Consequently, SDB prevalence in a cohort will change over time, and will vary across populations with differences in age and sex distribution, and in the proportion of overweight people. Of particular concern, adults and children in the United States and other countries are experiencing an increase in overweight and obesity.[28,29] With our longitudinal data over the past 20 years, we have observed an increase in body mass index (BMI) in the WSCS corresponding to national trends in the obesity epidemic. And, matching this epidemic, SDB prevalence has increased markedly.[27]

The Cost of Sleep-Disordered Breathing: Health Care Costs, Well-being, Morbidity, and Mortality

With cross-sectional data, we have explored the associations of SDB with hypertension, quality of life, motor vehicle accidents, and stroke.[7] Our analyses, controlling for potential confounding factors, have shown that SDB is associated with significant negative health outcomes, but the cross-sectional data limit a determination of what proportions of the outcomes are attributable to SDB. As our longitudinal data increase, we have been able to explore differences in incidence of some health outcomes by SDB status among those free of the specific outcome at baseline. The adverse outcomes predicted by SDB from longitudinal data, summarized in **Table 1**, provide better estimates for understanding the health and well-being burden that may be attributed to SDB (ie, likely to have a casual role).

Regardless of how blood pressure (BP) was measured, we have found significant associations between SDB and hypertension or elevated BP. With a prospective design, we excluded all WSCS participants who had existing hypertension (defined as measured BP>140/90 or using antihypertensive medication), and followed the group free of hypertension at baseline for 4 to 8 years to determine the incidence of new hypertension.[30] After controlling for age, sex, BMI, initial BP, and other confounding factors, we found a dose-response increased risk for developing hypertension with SDB. The 4-year incidence of hypertension was 2.9 greater for participants who had AHI greater than 15 versus less than 5 at baseline.

Using 24-hour ambulatory BP monitoring, we found participants who had SDB had higher BP levels before, during, and after sleep, compared with those who did not have SDB.[31] Longitudinally, we repeated ambulatory BP monitoring at 4-year intervals to determine the incidence of developing an abnormal nighttime BP pattern, described by the lack of 10% or greater dip in BP with sleep. This condition, referred to as "nondipping," has

been linked to poor prognosis for cardiovascular disease and death. We found SDB severity at baseline predicted an increase in the incidence of nondipping: participants who had AHI greater than 15 versus less than 5 at baseline had a fourfold greater odds of developing nondipping nocturnal BP.

Other longitudinal analyses of the WSCS data have linked SDB with the development of depression, measured by the Zung Self-Rating Depression Scale,[32] and incident stroke.[33] Most recently, we have assessed the 18-year mortality rate by SDB status at baseline. The rate of all-cause mortality was threefold higher for participants who had severe SDB, with AHI greater than 30, compared with those who did not have SDB.[26]

Longitudinal analyses with the WSCS data support the hypothesis that SDB has a role in increasing significant cardiovascular morbidity, depression, and mortality. After accounting for confounding factors, persons who had SDB, particularly severe, untreated SDB, had a three- to five-times greater incidence of the leading causes of poor health and well-being, and mortality. Corroboration from other population studies is needed, but our findings suggest that the burden of SDB is large because of a high prevalence of untreated SDB and potentially high attributable risk for significant adverse health and well-being outcomes.

Modifiers

Factors that alter the prevalence or the adverse consequences of SDB are important in determining the total societal burden. Identification of causal factors that have a direct role in initiating the development of SDB or that worsen progression may justify intervention programs only if the factors can be reduced. Body weight is an established risk factor for SDB.[6,7] Longitudinal analyses indicate weight is a modifiable risk factor.[34,35] Relative to stable weight over a 4-year period, a 10% loss in weight was associated with a decrease in SDB severity, as shown by a 23% reduction in AHI; a 10% gain in weight was associated with a sixfold (95% CI 2.2–17.0) greater risk for developing moderate or worse SDB, and a 32% increase in AHI progression.[34] As a modifiable risk factor, weight loss should hold the greatest promise as a means to reduce SDB prevalence. However, as a result of the ongoing strong trends in weight gain in both adults and children, the opposite result is likely: SDB prevalence is bound to increase. Using the relative risks from the WSCS analysis, and data on obesity trends

Table 1
Wisconsin Sleep Cohort Study: longitudinal associations of baseline sleep-disordered breathing with development of adverse health outcomes

Outcome	Follow-up Time (Mean)	Adjustment Variables	Odds ratio (95% confidence interval) for outcome and SDB severity level[a]	
			Moderate Versus None	Severe Versus None
Incident Hypertension[30] >140/90 mm Hg or use of antihypertensives	4 y	Age, sex, BMI, waist, hip girth, health hx, BP, smoking, alcohol	2.0 (1.2–3.2)	2.9 (1.5–5.6)
Incident "nondipping"[31] loss of ≥10% drop in systolic BP from wake to sleep	4 y	Age, sex, BMI, BP, smoking, alcohol, sleep duration, antihypertensive medications	3.1 (1.3–7.7)	4.4 (1.2–16.0)
Incident depression[32] Zung score>50	4 y	Age, sex, BMI, alcohol, education	2.0 (1.4–2.9)	2.6 (1.7–3.9)
Incident stroke[33]	4 y	Age, sex	n.s.	4.5 (1.3–15.0)
All-cause mortality[26]	14 y	Age, sex, BMI	n.s	3.0 (1.4–6.3)
All-cause mortality,[26] CPAP users excluded	14 s	Age, sex, BMI	n.s	3.8 (1.6–9.0)
Cardiovascular mortality,[26] CPAP users excluded	14 y	Age, sex, BMI	n.s	5.2 (1.4–19.0)

Abbreviations: BP, blood pressure; hx, history
  [a] No SDB was defined as AHI less than 5; moderate SDB was defined as AHI 5 to 15; and severe SDB was defined as AHI greater than 30 for mortality outcomes, AHI greater than 20 for stroke, and AHI greater than 15 for all other outcomes. Odds ratios were estimated with AHI less than 5 as the reference category.

and BMI distributions by age and sex in the United States between 1992 and 2008, we estimated that the prevalence of SDB would nearly double, and that the attributable proportion of SDB prevalence at a severity level of AHI greater than 15 would rise from 56% to 69% by 2008.[28]

Effective treatment of SDB is an extremely important modifier of the total social burden. It has been clear to clinicians within the field of sleep medicine that CPAP effectively prevented apnea and hypopnea episodes, and represented a significant way to reduce the adverse sequelae of SDB.[5] Consequently, if all SDB could be diagnosed and treated, the total burden would be equal to the direct cost of care for SDB, a small fraction of the potential burden of untreated SDB. However, in 1990, Wright[36] and others pointed out the lack of randomized trials of CPAP, and suggested that outside the field of sleep medicine, effective therapy for SDB was yet to be proved, which led to swift action in the sleep field to promote proposals for CPAP trials. Two ongoing, randomized, placebo-controlled clinical trials of CPAP (APPLES, centered at Stanford University[37] and CATNAP, centered at University of Pennsylvania[38]) will be critical to quantify the burden of SDB that can be reduced by treatment.

SUMMARY

In summary, findings from the WSCS and other population studies indicate

1. The first component of total social or public burden of SDB (see **Fig. 1**) poses a significant concern: The number of persons who have untreated SDB is large, with at least 12 to 18 million affected adults. Of additional concern, the prevalence will rise markedly on the coattails of the obesity epidemic. Similarly, as the population of the United States ages, the prevalence of SDB will increase because of the accumulation of cases and the likelihood that the incidence is higher in older age.
2. Limited longitudinal findings from the WSCS supporting a causal role of SDB in increased morbidity and mortality indicate that the second part of the total burden of SDB is significant. SDB is likely to contribute to increased cases of hypertension, cardiovascular disease, stroke, depression, and mortality. Adjusted relative risks and hazard ratios indicate moderate to large effect size (eg, **Table 1**, point estimates of risk for significant health outcomes with severe SDB range from 2.5–5).
3. The burden of SDB, reflected by the many persons who have this disorder multiplied by

the cost of adverse consequences that can be attributed to SDB, is likely to be staggering. The burden could be decreased by preventing SDB through risk factor reduction, with weight loss as the most likely candidate. However, national and international trends predict the opposite; it is unlikely that reduction in SDB prevalence and severity will occur in the near future. Modification of the total burden by diagnosis and treatment with CPAP holds the greatest hope for reduction of the SDB burden. Results from the forthcoming clinical trials on the proportion of SDB adverse effects that can be reduced with CPAP treatment will greatly increase our understanding of the burden of treated and untreated SDB. These data, in conjunction with (1) robust estimates of the number of affected people, according to age, sex, and other subgroups, and (2) the proportion of morbidity and mortality than can be attributed to SDB will provide a solid basis for developing appropriate health policy and its rapid translation to health care, to eventually reduce the total public burden of SDB.

REFERENCES

1. Colten H, Altevogt B, editors. Committee on sleep medicine and research, board on health sciences policy: sleep disorders and sleep deprivation: an unmet public health problem. Washington DC: Institute of Medicine/National Academies Press; 2006. p. 20–32.
2. Somers VK, White DP, Amin R, et al. Sleep apnea and cardiovascular disease. An American Heart Association/American College of Cardiology Foundation scientific statement. Circulation 2008;118:1080–111.
3. Namen AM, Dunagan DP, Fleischer A, et al. Increased physician-reported sleep apnea: the National ambulatory medical care survey. Chest 2002;121(6):1741–7.
4. Ball EM, Simon RD Jr, Tall AA, et al. Diagnosis and treatment of sleep apnea within the community. The Walla Walla project. Arch Intern Med 1997;157(4):419–24.
5. Shepard JW Jr, Buysse DJ, Chesson AL Jr, et al. History of the development of sleep medicine in the United States. J Clin Sleep Med 2005;1(1):61–82.
6. Punjabi NM. The epidemiology of adult obstructive sleep apnea. Proc Am Thorac Soc 2008;5:136–43.
7. Young T, Peppard PE, Gottlieb DJ, et al. Epidemiology of obstructive sleep apnea: a population health perspective. Am J Respir Crit Care Med 2002;165:1217–39.
8. Gislason T, Almqvist M, Eriksson G, et al. Prevalence of sleep apnea syndrome among Swedish men–an epidemiological study. J Clin Epidemiol 1988;41(6):571–6.
9. Bixler EO, Vgontzas AN, Ten Have T, et al. Effects of age on sleep apnea in men: I. Prevalence and severity. Am J Respir Crit Care Med 1998;157(1):144–8.

10. Bixler EO, Vgontzas AN, Lin HM, et al. Prevalence of sleep-disordered breathing in women: effects of gender. Am J Respir Crit Care Med 2001;163(3 Pt 1):608–13.

11. Lavie P. Incidence of sleep apnea in a presumably healthy working population: a significant relationship with excessive daytime sleepiness. Sleep 1983;6(4):312–8.

12. Bliwise DL, Bliwise NG, Partinen M, et al. Sleep apnea and mortality in an aged cohort. Am J Public Health 1988;78(5):544–7.

13. Bliwise D, Carskadon M, Carey E, et al. Longitudinal development of sleep-related respiratory disturbance in adult humans. J Gerontol 1984;39(3):290–3.

14. Ancoli-Israel S, Kripke DF, Mason W, et al. Characteristics of obstructive and central sleep apnea in the elderly: an interim report. Biol Psychiatry 1987;22(6):741–50.

15. Bliwise DL, Carey E, Dement WC, et al. Nightly variation in sleep-related respiratory disturbance in older adults. Exp Aging Res 1983;9(2):77–81.

16. Kryger MH. Sleep apnea. From the needles of Dionysius to continuous positive airway pressure. Arch Intern Med 1983;143(12):2301–3.

17. Lavie P. Who was the first to use the term Pickwickian in connection with sleepy patients? History of sleep apnoea syndrome. Sleep Med Rev 2008;12(1):5–17.

18. Gastaut H, Tassinari CA, Duron B, et al. Polygraphic study of the episodic diurnal and nocturnal (hypnic and respiratory) manifestations of the Pickwick syndrome. Brain Res 1966;1(2):167–86.

19. Sullivan CE, Issa FG, Berthon-Jones M, et al. Reversal of obstructive sleep apnoea by continuous positive airway pressure applied through the nares. Lancet 1981;1(8225):862–5.

20. National Commission on Sleep Disorders Research. Wake up America: a national sleep alert. Report of the National Commission on Sleep Disorders Research, 1993.

21. Kales A, Cadieux RJ, Bixler, et al. Severe obstructive sleep apnea–I: onset, clinical course, and characteristics. J Chronic Dis 1985;38(5):419–25.

22. Kales A, Caldwell AB, Cadieux RJ, et al. Severe obstructive sleep apnea–II: associated psychopathology and psychosocial consequences. J Chronic Dis 1985;38(5):427–34.

23. Gislason T, Taube A. Prevalence of sleep apnea syndrome–estimation by two stage sampling. Ups J Med Sci 1987;92(2):193–203.

24. Young T, Palta M, Dempsey J, et al. The occurrence of sleep-disordered breathing among middle-aged adults. N Engl J Med 1993;328:1230–5.

25. Young T, Hutton R, Finn L, et al. The gender bias in sleep apnea diagnosis. Are women missed because they have different symptoms? Arch Intern Med 1995;156:2445–51.

26. Young T, Finn L, Peppard PE, et al. Sleep disordered breathing and mortality: eighteen-year follow-up of the Wisconsin sleep Cohort. Sleep 2008;31(8):1071–8.

27. Young T, Peppard PE, Taheri S, et al. Excess weight and sleep-disordered breathing. J Appl Phys 2005;99(4):1592–9.

28. Prentice AM. The emerging epidemic of obesity in developing countries. Int J Epidemiol 2006;35(1):93–9.

29. Hedley AA, Ogden CL, Johnson CL, et al. Prevalence of overweight and obesity among US children, adolescents, and adults, 1999–2002. JAMA 2004;291(23):2847–50.

30. Peppard PE, Young T, Palta M, et al. Prospective study of the association between sleep-disordered breathing and hypertension. N Engl J Med 2000;342:1378–84.

31. Hla KM, Young T, Finn L, et al. Longitudinal association of sleep-disordered breathing and nondipping of nocturnal blood pressure in the Wisconsin sleep Cohort study. Sleep 2008;31(6):795–800.

32. Arzt M, Young T, Finn L, et al. Association of sleep-disordered breathing and the occurrence of stroke. Am J Respir Crit Care Med 2005;172:1447–51.

33. Peppard PE, Szklo-Coxe M, Hla KM, et al. Longitudinal association of sleep-related breathing disorder and depression. Arch Intern Med 2006;166(16):1709–15.

34. Peppard PE, Young T, Palta M, et al. Longitudinal study of moderate weight change and sleep-disordered breathing. JAMA 2000;284(23):3015–21.

35. Newman AB, Foster G, Givelber R, et al. Progression and regression of sleep-disordered breathing with changes in weight: the sleep heart health study. Arch Intern Med 2005;165(20):2408–13.

36. Wright J, Johns R, Watt I, et al. Health effects of obstructive sleep apnoea and the effectiveness of continuous positive airways pressure: a systematic review of the research evidence. BMJ 1997;314(7084):851–60.

37. Kushida CA, Nichols DA, Quan SF, et al. The Apnea positive pressure long-term efficacy study (APPLES): rationale, design, methods, and procedures. J Clin Sleep Med 2006;2(3):288–300.

38. Weaver TE, Maislin G, Dinges DF, et al. Relationship between hours of CPAP use and achieving normal levels of sleepiness and daily functioning. Sleep 2007;30(6):711–9.

Epidemiology of Sleep-Disordered Breathing: Lessons from the Sleep Heart Health Study

Naresh M. Punjabi, MD, PhD[a],*, R. Nisha Aurora, MD[b]

KEYWORDS

- Sleep-disordered breathing • Sleep apnea
- Cardiovascular disease • Hypertension

Sleep-disordered breathing (SDB) is a chronic condition that is characterized by partial or complete collapse of the upper airway during sleep. The resulting apneas and hypopneas lead to a reduction in oxyhemoglobin saturation and recurrent arousals from sleep. Aside from the obvious complaints of daytime fatigue and excessive sleepiness, SDB is associated with impaired cognitive function, poor work performance, increased risk for motor vehicle accidents, and a constellation of problems in daily living that diminish quality of life.[1,2] Although the clinical syndrome of SDB has been known for decades, it was not until 1988 that the National Commission of Sleep Disorders Research was established by Congress to address the public health importance of SDB and other sleep-related disorders. In 1993, the commission issued a comprehensive report that set forth key research priorities for the field of sleep medicine with the specific acknowledgment that coordinated efforts were needed to define the health-related effects of SDB. At about the same time, the potential morbidity and mortality associated with even moderate severity of SDB were being increasingly recognized, and the means to diagnose the condition efficiently were becoming readily available. Shortly thereafter, newly available data on the population prevalence of SDB revealed that millions of Americans were affected by this condition, with most being undiagnosed.[3,4] Given the epidemic of obesity and its strong association with SDB, a major initiative was set forth by the National Institutes of Health to define the public health impact of SDB. The Sleep Heart Health Study (SHHS), a product of that initiative, was established to answer many of the pressing questions regarding the clinical consequences of SDB, particularly its effects on hypertension and cardiovascular disease. The primary objective of this article is to review briefly the scientific progress made by the SHHS over the last decade. Within the context of this nonexhaustive review of the SHHS, some of the most pivotal findings available to date are highlighted. However, before discussing these findings, the design and recruitment strategies are reviewed, along with the major clinical end points of interest.

DESIGN OF THE SLEEP HEART HEALTH STUDY

The SHHS is a multicenter cohort study sponsored by the National Heart, Lung, and Blood Institute to assess the cardiovascular and noncardiovascular consequences of SDB.[5] This study was motivated by the increasing recognition that SDB was

Supported by National Institutes of Health Grants HL075078 and HL086862.

[a] Division of Pulmonary and Critical Care Medicine, Department of Medicine, Johns Hopkins University School of Medicine, 5501 Hopkins Bayview Circle, Baltimore, MD 21224, USA

[b] Division of Pulmonary, Critical Care, and Sleep Medicine, One Gustave L. Levy Place, Box 1232, Mount Sinai School of Medicine, New York, NY 10029, USA

* Corresponding author. Division of Pulmonary and Critical Care Medicine, Johns Hopkins University School of Medicine, 5501 Hopkins Bayview Circle, Baltimore, MD 21224, USA.

E-mail address: npunjabi@jhmi.edu (N.M. Punjabi).

prevalent in the general population and that it may increase the risk for several cardiovascular conditions, including hypertension, coronary artery disease, and stroke. To maximize efficiency, the SHHS drew on the resources of existing, well-characterized, epidemiologic cohorts, and conducted further data collection, including nocturnal measurements of sleep and breathing patterns. These cohorts included the Framingham Offspring and Omni Cohort Studies, the Atherosclerosis Risk in Communities Study, the Cardiovascular Health Study, the Strong Heart Study, the Tucson Epidemiologic Study of Respiratory Disease, and the New York City Studies on hypertension. Details regarding individual cohorts have been published previously.[5]

The decision to recruit from established cohort studies instead of starting with a new cohort was motivated by several advantages associated with the former approach. First, recruiting from other studies was cost effective and obviated the burden of recruiting a large sample from the general community. Second, aside from measures of SDB, data on essential covariates and health outcomes were being collected by each of the "parent" studies as part of their local data collection process. Thus, by adding on nocturnal polysomnography, participant burden was increased only by a limited degree to address fundamental questions on the clinical relevance of SDB. Third, access to relevant cardiovascular risk factors before the initiation of the SHHS conferred a unique opportunity to examine how prevalent medical conditions would modify SDB-related end points. Finally, using established cohorts increased the probability of enrollment and retention of a study sample that would need to be followed for more than a decade. Thus, between 1995 and 1997, a sample of 6441 participants was recruited from the above "parent" studies. Participants younger than 65 years of age were oversampled on self-reported snoring to augment the prevalence of SDB. Enrollment had no upper age limit and prevalent cardiovascular disease was not an exclusionary criterion. In addition to the in-home polysomnogram, extensive data on usual sleep habits, resting blood pressure, body composition measures (eg, body mass index [BMI], waist circumference, neck circumference), prescription and nonprescription medication use, daytime sleep tendency (eg, Epworth Sleepiness Scale [ESS]), and quality of life were also collected. Outcomes assessments were coordinated to provide standardized information on hypertension and incident cardiovascular events, including myocardial infarction, coronary revascularization, congestive heart failure, and stroke. As part of

this first large-scale effort to characterize sleep and breathing abnormalities in the community, new methods for data collection were needed, along with new approaches to minimize between-site differences in overnight monitoring. In addition, protocols for centralized scoring of sleep and breathing abnormalities were developed. In the following section, techniques for in-home polysomnography that were used in the SHHS are discussed in conjunction with issues regarding central assessment of the sleep recordings.

UNATTENDED HOME POLYSOMNOGRAPHY

Given the recruitment of subjects from several geographic sites, methods were needed to assure uniform data collection and analysis. In contrast to the laboratory-based methods, the SHHS opted to conduct home polysomnography. Recording sleep in the home was deemed to be the most convenient method to minimize participant burden and study cost, given the large number of subjects located across different cities. In choosing a methodology for sleep recordings, several constraints were considered, such as the capability of capturing several physiologic signals while balancing convenience and portability. In selecting the equipment, 13 different systems were evaluated that met the minimal criteria set forth by the SHHS leadership. From this set of 13 systems, 1 was selected that included a data acquisition recorder with a rechargeable battery that could allow approximately 15 hours of recording. Digital information collected by the recorder was stored on an internal memory card that could be accessed for downloading the sleep recordings.

The recording montage included the following channels: C_3-A_2 and C_4-A_1 electroencephalograms (EEG), right and left electro-oculograms (EOG), a single bipolar electrocardiogram, chin electromyogram (EMG), oxyhemoglobin saturation by pulse oximetry, chest and abdominal excursion by inductance plethysmography, airflow by an oronasal thermocouple, and body position by a mercury gauge. The EEG data were collected at a sampling rate of 125 Hz. All sleep recordings were stored in real time on internal memory cards that were then transferred to erasable digital media and shipped to a central reading center for review. Sleep stage scoring at the reading center was performed by trained technicians according to the criteria of Rechtschaffen and Kales.[6] Scoring of breathing abnormalities was conducted as follows: Apneas were identified if thermocouple airflow was absent or nearly absent for at least 10 seconds. Hypopneas were identified if discernible reductions in thermocouple airflow or thoracoabdominal movement (at least 30% below baseline values) occurred for at least 10 seconds. The respiratory disturbance index (RDI) was defined as the number of apneas or hypopneas, each associated with a 4% decrease in oxygen saturation, per hour of sleep.[7] Arousals were identified as abrupt shifts of at least 3 seconds' duration in EEG frequency. For rapid eye movement (REM) sleep, scoring of arousals also required concurrent increases in EMG amplitude.[8] An arousal index was defined as the average number of arousals per hour of sleep.

One of the major challenges for the SHHS was to assess the variability of sleep data acquired across the different sites. Assessments of study quality showed that approximately 48% of the sleep studies were rated as excellent or outstanding, 39% were rated as good or very good, and 13% were rated as fair. Adequate data were not initially obtained in 9.4% of the sample.[9] However, after a repeat attempt, the effective failure rate dropped to 5.3%. Quality grades were best for the EOG recordings, followed by the EEG and EMG channels. More than 4 hours of artifact-free EEG and EOG data were collected in 90% and 98% of the studies, respectively. For each of the other channels (ie, EMG, thermocouple, chest band, abdomen band), more than 85% of the studies had more than 4 hours of artifact-free data. Analysis of associations between study quality grade and factors such as age, gender, BMI, and SDB severity showed that the impact of these factors on quality was negligible.[10] Thus, despite the challenges of monitoring sleep in an unattended setting, the SHHS data show that, with proper methodology and adequate training, complex physiologic data can be collected reliably in the home setting on a large community sample.

While it was essential to standardize the collection of sleep data, it was also imperative that the recordings be interpreted reliably if meaningful associations were to be uncovered between metrics of SDB and cardiovascular outcomes. To determine intra- and interscorer reliability of scoring sleep and respiratory events, a subset of studies with good or better overall quality was chosen at random for examination.[11] For sleep staging, interscorer reliability comparisons showed kappa statistics in the range of 0.81 to 0.83. When sleep stages were assessed as wake, non-REM sleep, and REM sleep, the interscorer agreement increased with kappa statistics in the 0.87 to 0.90 range. The interscorer reliability of scoring respiratory events was also high, with intraclass correlation coefficients of 0.99 for the RDI based on either a 4% or 5% oxyhemoglobin

desaturation criterion. However, the reliability in scoring EEG arousals was modest, with an intraclass correlation of 0.54. These analyses demonstrate that, with rigorous training and proper oversight, a high degree of inter- and intrascorer reliability can be achieved for scoring of sleep stages and disordered breathing events.

Having shown that polysomnographic data can be collected systematically in the home setting and scored reliably, it was important to determine the existence of any significant night-to-night variability in sleep stages, arousal frequency, and the RDI.[12] A high degree of variability in these measures could potentially jeopardize the ability to identify relevant associations with clinical outcomes that are to be ascertained years, or even decades later, after the baseline sleep assessment. Fortunately, in a sample of subjects who had repeat polysomnograms approximately 2 months apart (average 77 days, range 31–112 days), no significant differences were observed in the sleep efficiency, arousal index, or distribution of sleep stages. Furthermore, no bias was noted in the RDI between the two sleep studies. In a distinct study sample, comparisons were also undertaken to determine whether the sleep recordings in the home would systematically differ from those derived in an attended laboratory setting. These analyses showed that, compared with the laboratory, home recordings had a higher median sleep duration (375 versus 318 minutes; $P<0.0001$) and a higher sleep efficiency (86% versus 82%; $P<.0024$). Although differences existed in the RDI, they were small. Taken together, these studies show that unsupervised home monitoring provides an accurate and stable assessment of sleep architecture and SDB when compared with that acquired in a clinical sleep laboratory. With that background on methodology, the sections that follow cover a range of topics based on some of the primary findings from the SHHS. These include: (1) clinical predictors of SDB; (2) impact of SDB on daytime sleepiness; (3) SDB-related impairment in quality of life; and (4) associations between SDB, hypertension, cardiovascular disease, and metabolic dysfunction.

CLINICAL PREDICTORS OF SLEEP-DISORDERED BREATHING

Initial reports on potential risk factors for SDB in patient populations showed that older age, male sex, central obesity, and habitual snoring were independently associated with the presence and severity of SDB. Although these reports pioneered the efforts of identifying those at risk, most were not generalizable to nonclinical samples, given that the analyses were often based on patients referred for clinical symptoms. Subsequently, several community- and population-based studies revealed that some of the earlier observations on the clinical correlates of SDB were not representative and could not be applied to the general population. For example, in clinic-based samples, SDB was noted to be 8 to 10 times more likely in men than women. However, in the general community, it was noted that men are only 2 to 3 times more likely to have SDB than women.[13] Thus, such data would suggest an inherent referral bias in clinical samples, and that case identification of SDB in women is disproportionately lower than the true burden of disease. To further assess factors associated with SDB in a community sample, the SHHS data were plumbed to quantify the relative importance of age, sex, race, obesity, self-reported snoring, and breathing pauses during sleep as potential predictors.[14] These analyses showed that although male sex was an independent risk factor, the odds ratio for moderate-to-severe SDB (defined as an RDI $\geq$ 15 events/h) comparing men and women was approximately 1.5, an estimate in line with those derived from studies using nonclinical samples. Furthermore, obesity, and in particular central obesity, was also correlated with SDB. Analysis of BMI, neck circumference, and waist-to-hip ratio revealed that BMI and neck circumference were independently correlated with prevalent SDB. In contrast, waist-to-hip ratio provided no additional predictive value after the inclusion of BMI and neck circumference. The odds ratios for prevalent SDB associated with a one standard deviation increment in BMI and neck circumference were approximately 1.5 and 1.6, respectively. Contrary to previous work, subjects of a minority race (eg, African Americans and American Indians) were comparable to their white counterparts in the prevalence of SDB after accounting for factors such as age, sex, BMI, and neck circumference. This finding raises the question of whether demographic and anthropometric factors explain the previously documented excess risk for SDB in minority populations. Finally, self-reported habitual snoring, the intensity of the snoring, and frequently observed apneas were independently predictive of SDB. Reports of habitual snoring had better predictive value for SDB in women than in men and witnessed apneas were more predictive of SDB in younger versus older subjects.

An additional and important contribution of the cross-sectional analysis was the demonstration that SDB prevalence increases with age. Although a linear association between age and SDB prevalence had been suggested previously, the SHHS data showed that the prevalence does increase linearly with age, but only until the sixth decade. Thereafter, the prevalence of moderate-to-severe SDB reaches a relative plateau for those in the seventh and eighth decades. Age modified the effects of body composition and self-reported snoring and breathing pauses on the prevalence of SDB. In each case, the effect was attenuated with increasing age, suggesting that obesity and symptoms of snoring and breathing pauses are poor predictors of SDB in the older population.

Although the clinical factors associated with SDB discussed in this section are relevant to case identification and risk stratification, perhaps the most common complaint that leads patients who have SDB to seek medical attention is excessive daytime sleepiness. The next section focuses on this specific consequence of SDB.

SLEEP-DISORDERED BREATHING AND EXCESSIVE DAYTIME SLEEPINESS

Recurrent apneas and hypopneas disrupt sleep continuity and thus infringe on the restorative function of sleep. Whether sleepiness is assessed objectively (eg, multiple sleep latency test) or subjectively (eg, ESS), patients who have SDB are generally sleepier than normal subjects. Despite this well-established effect, the SHHS data have provided a unique view of the association between SDB severity and the degree of daytime impairment in a nonclinical sample. Confirming previous work, the severity of SDB was directly correlated with the degree of daytime sleepiness.[15] The percentage of subjects who had excessive sleepiness, defined as an ESS score of at least 11, increased from 21% in those who did not have SDB (RDI<5 events/h) to 35% in those who had moderate-to-severe SDB (RDI $\geq$ 30 events/h). The mean ESS score increased monotonically with disease severity from 7.2 (RDI < 5 events/h) to 9.3 (RDI $\geq$ 30 events/h). The relationship between SDB and excessive sleep tendency was not modified by factors such as age, sex, BMI, or sleep duration. Furthermore, analyses that included snoring and the RDI as covariates in multivariable statistical models showed that both of these variables were independently associated with excessive sleepiness. Even in those subjects who did not have SDB, snoring frequency correlated directly with the ESS score. For example, in subjects who had an RDI of less than 1.5 events/h, the average ESS score was 6.1 in never-snorers and increased to an average of 8.8 in habitual snorers. Whether snoring is a mere proxy for disordered breathing events that were not captured within the RDI or whether snoring can fragment sleep continuity and lead to excessive sleepiness remains to be determined. Having described the impact of SDB on excessive sleepiness, the question of whether SDB is associated with impaired quality of life is discussed next.

SLEEP-DISORDERED BREATHING AND QUALITY OF LIFE

The quality and quantity of sleep can have a considerable impact on overall quality of life. Although the definition of quality of life is still a topic of significant debate, it is a subjective concept which refers to how an individual perceives his or her level of daily functioning. Quality of life is a multidimensional construct that represents a sum of a person's physical, emotional, psychologic, and social well-being. The term "health-related quality of life" is a subset of the overall concept of quality of life and is used as a means of characterizing the patient's subjective experience of health and disease. The science of measuring health-related quality of life has advanced sufficiently and new instruments are constantly added to the already existing armamentarium of available measures. Health status instruments can be classified as either generic or disease specific. Generic health-related quality of life instruments are designed to quantify the impairments in various dimensions of health status imposed by a disease process. The advantages of such instruments include their broad scope, the availability of normative data, and the ability to compare different conditions. The 36-Item Short Form Health Survey (SF-36) is one such self-administered generic quality of life instrument that has gained much popularity over the last decade. It consists of eight dimensions, which include physical functioning, social functioning, role physical, bodily pain, mental health, role emotional, vitality, and general health. Scores for each dimension or subscale range from 0 to 100, with higher scores representing a better quality of life.

The extent to which the SDB, difficulty initiating and maintaining sleep (DIMS), and self-reported excessive sleepiness are associated with impairments in quality of life has been explored using the baseline data from the SHHS.[16] Although these analyses replicate previous work,[17] they also provide new and unique insights. First, women were more likely to report symptoms of DIMS than men, whereas men were more likely to have SDB than women. Second, severe SDB (RDI $\geq$ 30 events/h), DIMS, and excessive

sleepiness (ESS $\geq$ 11) were associated with impaired quality of life as evidenced by lower SF-36 scores on most of its subscales. Third, a linear association was noted between vitality and the degree of SDB severity, an effect that did not vary between men and women. Finally, excessive daytime sleepiness was also negatively correlated with each of the SF-36 subscales. For example, men reporting excessive sleepiness (ESS score $\geq$ 11) had a 1.83 higher odds for having a lower mental health score compared with men who did not have excessive sleepiness (ESS score < 11). Although a similar effect was observed in women, the strength of association was not as large (odds ratio 1.31), indicating effect modification by sex. Perhaps one of the most important aspects of this work is that it also compared SDB and other sleep symptoms to other chronic medical conditions with regard to their impact on quality of life. These comparisons showed that SDB and excessive sleepiness not only impair quality of life but do so to the same extent as conditions such as hypertension and diabetes mellitus. Although much remains to be delineated with regards to the additive and interactive effects of SDB-related comorbidities on quality of life, those who have SDB suffer obvious impairments in their daily living.

SLEEP-DISORDERED BREATHING AND HYPERTENSION

One of the most controversial issues in sleep medicine is whether SDB is an independent risk factor for systemic hypertension. The debate over a causal association stems from the fact that both disorders share common antecedent factors, including male sex, obesity, and older age. Although initial reports failed to account for these confounders, accumulating evidence over the past decade supports the hypothesis that SDB and its associated pathophysiologic consequences contribute to the development of systemic hypertension. Acute consequences of SDB on nocturnal blood pressure have been well characterized.[18] Brief upper airway occlusion (apnea or hypopnea) during sleep is typically associated with a fall in arterial oxygen tension and a concomitant rise in systemic blood pressure. The peak in blood pressure occurs shortly after termination of the apnea. The apnea-related surge in blood pressure has been attributed to the activation of the sympathetic nervous system by several factors, including hypoxemia, hypercapnia, changes in intrathoracic pressure, and arousal from sleep. Although hypoxemia and arousal appear to be primary determinants of the acute hemodynamic response related to an obstructive event, the relative contribution of these two factors to the development of systemic hypertension is not known. Experimental data from animal models show that hypoxia is a potent stimulus for activating the sympathetic nervous system and thus may increase blood pressure.[19] However, data from other experimental studies indicate that apnea-related arousals can also contribute to the acute elevation of arterial pressure.[20]

Despite the fact that experimental short-term studies have provided mechanistic insight into the increase in blood pressure associated with apneas and hypopnea, the relative importance of SDB as a causal factor for systemic hypertension needs to be defined in clinical studies. Early reports revealed that 30% to 50% of patients who had SDB had systemic hypertension and that 30% to 50% of patients who had systemic hypertension had SDB.[21] However, as with many clinic-based studies, appropriate adjustments for confounding were either absent or provided conflicting results. Moreover, a relative paucity on community- or population-based data on whether the association would hold true in nonclinical samples exists. Thus, the cross-sectional analysis of the SHHS data filled some of gaps in the existing literature.[22] Prevalent hypertension was defined as a blood pressure of at least 140/90 or current treatment with an antihypertensive medication. Primary findings from these analyses showed that mean systolic and diastolic blood pressure and the prevalence of hypertension increased directly with measures of SDB including the RDI and measures of nocturnal hypoxemia. These associations were present in both sexes, in older and younger subjects, and across all ethnic groups. Perhaps the most striking was the finding of a higher odds ratio for hypertension in subjects who had even mild SDB (RDI 5.0–14.9 events/h).

Corroborating these findings, the Wisconsin Sleep Cohort[23,24] and the Penn Sleep Cohort[25] studies have also shown a cross-sectional and an independent association between SDB and hypertension. Over the last several years, longitudinal data from the Wisconsin Sleep Cohort Study have provided additional evidence that SDB is associated with incident hypertension.[26] Reproducibility of the associations across different epidemiologic cohorts coupled with robust clinical trial data on the favorable effects of positive airway pressure therapy on blood pressure make a compelling argument that SDB is a risk factor for systemic hypertension. It is hoped that ongoing follow-up from the SHHS will add to this growing body of evidence and substantiate the notion that SDB can influence blood pressure, and thus justify case identification and early intervention for this disorder in the general community. Deriving unequivocal evidence for the impact of SDB on hypertension is essential, given that it is a precursor for cardiovascular disease. Thus, as discussed in the following section, SDB could also mediate cardiovascular outcomes by increasing blood pressure and perhaps by other independent pathways.

SLEEP-DISORDERED BREATHING AND CARDIOVASCULAR DISEASE

Repetitive cycles of intermittent hypoxemia and sleep fragmentation provide an enriched physiologic milieu which, if sustained over time, could increase cardiovascular risk in people who have SDB. Putative intermediates that have been implicated in the genesis of SDB-related cardiovascular disease include heightened sympathetic nervous system activity, endothelial dysfunction, hypercoagulability, and an increase in oxidative stress and systemic inflammation. Perhaps acting synergistically, these pathophysiologic alterations can contribute to, or accelerate, the progression of various cardiovascular conditions such as coronary artery disease, myocardial infarction, heart failure, and stroke. Although several clinical case series and case-control studies have shown an association between SDB and cardiovascular diseases, large-scale epidemiologic studies using nonclinical samples are limited. Cross-sectional evidence from the SHHS indicates that the prevalence of coronary heart disease, heart failure, and stroke is higher in people with SDB than people without SDB.[27] Modeling prevalent cardiovascular disease as a function of the RDI showed that the adjusted odds ratios for the four RDI quartiles were 1.00 (RDI<1.3 events/h; first quartile); 0.98 (RDI 1.4–4.4 events/h; second quartile), 1.28 (RDI 4.5–11.0 events/h) and 1.42 (RDI>11.0 events/h; fourth quartile). Comparing the upper and lowest quartiles, SDB was most strongly associated with prevalent heart failure (odds ratio 2.38), followed by prevalent stroke (odds ratio 1.58), and coronary heart disease (odds ratio 1.27). These results indicate that even with mild disease, SDB may predispose to adverse cardiovascular outcomes. Obviously, causal cardiovascular implications cannot be assessed based on cross-sectional data. It is certainly possible that the observed associations in the SHHS and other studies are a result of reverse causality, and it is the presence of cardiovascular disease that is the predisposing factor for SDB. If a prospective association is indeed identified with longitudinal data from the SHHS and other cohorts, it would complement the recent findings from a large clinical series that showed that treatment with positive pressure therapy, at least in men who have severe SDB, can mitigate the risk for fatal and nonfatal cardiovascular events.[28]

Central to any discussion of cardiovascular disease and potential risk factors is the putative role of altered glucose metabolism. Understanding the significance of SDB for normal glucose homeostasis is clinically relevant because SDB could increase the risk for type 2 diabetes mellitus and, in turn, for future cardiovascular disease. Thus, in the next section, the authors describe the findings from the SHHS pertaining to its independent association with altered glucose metabolism.

SLEEP-DISORDERED BREATHING, INSULIN RESISTANCE, AND GLUCOSE INTOLERANCE

Numerous population- and clinic-based reports have suggested a possible link between SDB and altered glucose metabolism. As summarized in several comprehensive articles on this topic,[29,30] initial studies frequently used surrogate measures, especially snoring, to assess the presence of SDB. Additionally, metabolic assessments in these studies varied and included measures such as self-reported diabetes, fasting blood glucose and insulin levels, glucose tolerance tests, and glycosylated hemoglobin levels. Lack of adequate control for confounders, especially central obesity, limited interpretation of results from some of the earlier studies. The association between SDB, glucose intolerance, and insulin resistance has also been examined in the SHHS. For this analysis, SDB was characterized using the RDI, along with measurements of oxyhemoglobin desaturation during sleep.[31] Metabolic function was assessed with a glucose tolerance test and fasting levels of serum glucose and insulin. Confounding variables considered in these analyses included age, sex, smoking status, BMI, waist circumference, and sleep duration. This cross-sectional analysis demonstrated several relevant findings. First, a positive and significant dose–response relationship was noted between SDB severity, and fasting and 2-hour glucose levels. Second, subjects who had moderate-to-severe SDB (RDI $\geq$ 15 events/h) were noted to have higher values on the homeostasis model assessment index (HOMA), a product of fasting glucose and insulin values, indicating an insulin-resistant state independent of other factors. Third, average oxyhemoglobin saturation during sleep and percentage of sleep time below an oxyhemoglobin saturation of 90% were independently correlated with fasting hyperglycemia,

glucose intolerance, and the HOMA index of insulin resistance. Finally, although the arousal frequency was not correlated with glycemic status, it was associated with the HOMA index. Thus, the results of this analysis confirm the findings of previous clinic-based studies suggesting an independent relation between SDB and glucose dysregulation. Major strengths of this work include objective means for assessing SDB and metabolic function, adjustment for factors such as obesity, and the use of a nonclinical sample. These data also implicate sleep-related hypoxemia and possibly arousals as putative intermediates in the causal chain between SDB and metabolic dysfunction.

SLEEP DURATION, IMPAIRED GLUCOSE TOLERANCE, AND DIABETES MELLITUS

Although much of the foregoing discussion has focused on the lessons learned on the associates between SDB and various health outcomes, it is also imperative to highlight some of the work on how habitually short sleep duration, a pervasive problem in industrialized nations, correlates with health outcomes. Based on the annual polls conducted by the National Sleep Foundation, it is increasingly obvious that curtailment of habitual sleep duration is becoming one of the most prevalent sleep-related problems, as evidenced by a significant decline in the median sleep time of adults in the United States, from 8 hours per night in 1959 to less than 7 hours per night by 2002. Although less than 15% of adults in the United States reported sleeping fewer than 7 hours per night in 1959, by 2002 more than one-third were sleeping fewer than 7 hours per night. A rising number of developed and developing countries are moving toward a 24/7 lifestyle to meet the escalating demands for efficiency and productivity. Although the health consequences of being an "around-the-clock" society are not fully elucidated, voluntary sleep curtailment and its ensuing problems are becoming increasingly recognized. Neurocognitive impairments secondary to short habitual sleep duration are well recognized. Initial epidemiologic evidence suggesting a potential role for sleep duration in metabolic dysfunction came from the Nurses' Health Study, which demonstrated a higher incidence of diabetes in subjects reporting fewer than 6 hours or more than 9 hours of sleep 10 years after the assessment of sleep duration.[32] Experimental data provide additional support for the notion that short sleep duration may be associated with metabolic dysfunction. Healthy, nonobese, young adults subjected to 4 hours of sleep per night for 6 nights were noted to have approximately a 30% reduction in glucose tolerance.[33] Although this study showed acute effect of severe sleep restriction, it raised the possibility of a likely causal association between habitually short sleep duration and impaired glucose regulation.

The association of habitual sleep duration, impaired glucose tolerance, and diabetes was also examined in the SHHS cohort. Impaired glucose tolerance and diabetes in the SHHS were based on objective data, including fasting glucose values or the glucose tolerance test. The cross-sectional analysis of the SHHS corroborated previous epidemiologic evidence on this topic. Specifically, compared with subjects reporting sleeping 7 to 8 hours per night, those reporting 5 hours or fewer and 6 hours per night had adjusted odds ratios for prevalent diabetes of 2.51 and 1.66, respectively. The respective adjusted odds for prevalent impaired glucose tolerance were 1.33 and 1.58. Subjects sleeping 9 hours or more per night were also observed to have higher odds ratios for prevalent diabetes and impaired glucose tolerance. These results substantiate the findings from the Nurses' Health Study while accounting for several confounding variables that were not previously considered, including objective measures of SDB. The identification of an independent association provide the necessary platform on which additional human and animal investigations can be based to substantiate causality and define putative mechanisms. Additional research between short sleep duration and metabolic impairment is vital, given the ever-increasing prevalence of type 2 diabetes mellitus.

SLEEP DURATION AND HYPERTENSION

In addition to the noted association between sleep duration and metabolic impairment, the SHHS also provides supportive data on the relationship between sleep duration and hypertension. Although short-term experimental sleep restriction has been shown to increase blood pressure,[34,35] epidemiologic evidence supporting an association between sleep duration and hypertension is limited. In the SHHS cohort, sleep duration was ascertained with a sleep habits questionnaire, and hypertension was identified on the basis of measured blood pressure or the use of antihypertensive medication. Compared with subjects reporting sleeping on average 7 to 8 hours per night, those who had fewer than 7 hours per night or more than 8 hours per night had a higher prevalence of hypertension even after accounting for factors including age, sex, race, RDI, and obesity.

In a set of secondary analyses that included adjustments for other factors, such as caffeine and alcohol consumption, smoking, sleep efficiency, symptoms of insomnia and depression, prevalent diabetes mellitus, and prevalent cardiovascular disease, the odds ratio for hypertension for subjects reporting fewer than 6 hours of sleep was 1.66 compared with those reporting 7 to 8 hours of habitual sleep. Defining the role of habitual sleep duration in the development of hypertension is important because it could certainly increase the predisposition for overall cardiovascular morbidity and mortality.

FUTURE DIRECTIONS

The SHHS has provided a unique opportunity to better define the public health implications of SDB and sleep duration. During the first 10 years of this study, it has imparted many unique contributions to the field of sleep medicine. In particular, correlations between SDB and excessive daytime sleepiness, quality of life, hypertension, altered glucose metabolism, and cardiovascular disease have been elucidated in a large community cohort of middle-aged and older adults. Although causal links cannot necessarily be ascertained from the cross-sectional data published thus far, ongoing longitudinal analyses will help describe causal effects and better portray the natural history of SDB. It is essential that we gain a better understanding of the health burden associated with SDB and short sleep duration so as to implement strategies to curtail the clinical, economic, and societal costs encumbered by those undiagnosed with these conditions. Additionally, future findings from the SHHS will be critical in opening new avenues of sleep research and answering pressing questions concerning biologic mechanisms.

REFERENCES

1. Young T, Peppard PE, Gottlieb DJ. Epidemiology of obstructive sleep apnea: a population health perspective. Am J Respir Crit Care Med 2002;165: 1217–39.
2. Brown WD. The psychosocial aspects of obstructive sleep apnea. Semin Respir Crit Care Med 2005;26: 33–43.
3. Young T, Palta M, Dempsey J, et al. The occurrence of sleep-disordered breathing among middle-aged adults. N Engl J Med 1993;328:1230–5.
4. Young T, Evans L, Finn L, et al. Estimation of the clinically diagnosed proportion of sleep apnea syndrome in middle-aged men and women. Sleep 1997;20:705–6.

5. Quan SF, Howard BV, Iber C, et al. The Sleep Heart Health Study: design, rationale, and methods. Sleep 1997;20:1077–85.

6. Rechtschaffen A, Kales A. Manual of standardized terminology, techniques and scoring system for sleep stages of human subjects. Washington, DC: US Government Printing Office; 1968.

7. Sleep-related breathing disorders in adults: recommendations for syndrome definition and measurement techniques in clinical research. The report of an American Academy of Sleep Medicine Task Force. Sleep 1999;22:667–89.

8. EEG arousals: scoring rules and examples: a preliminary report from the Sleep Disorders Atlas Task Force of the American Sleep Disorders Association. Sleep 1992;15:173–84.

9. Redline S, Sanders MH, Lind BK, et al. Methods for obtaining and analyzing unattended polysomnography data for a multicenter study. Sleep Heart Health Research Group. Sleep 1998;21:759–67.

10. Kapur VK, Rapoport DM, Sanders MH, et al. Rates of sensor loss in unattended home polysomnography: the influence of age, gender, obesity, and sleep-disordered breathing. Sleep 2000;23:682–8.

11. Whitney CW, Gottlieb DJ, Redline S, et al. Reliability of scoring respiratory disturbance indices and sleep staging. Sleep 1998;21:749–57.

12. Quan SF, Griswold ME, Iber C, et al. Short-term variability of respiration and sleep during unattended nonlaboratory polysomnography–the Sleep Heart Health Study. Sleep 2002;25:843–9.

13. Redline S, Strohl KP. Recognition and consequences of obstructive sleep apnea hypopnea syndrome. Clin Chest Med 1998;19:1–19.

14. Young T, Shahar E, Nieto FJ, et al. Predictors of sleep-disordered breathing in community-dwelling adults: the Sleep Heart Health Study. Arch Intern Med 2002;162:893–900.

15. Gottlieb DJ, Whitney CW, Bonekat WH, et al. Relation of sleepiness to respiratory disturbance index: the Sleep Heart Health Study. Am J Respir Crit Care Med 1999;159:502–7.

16. Baldwin CM, Griffith KA, Nieto FJ, et al. The association of sleep-disordered breathing and sleep symptoms with quality of life in the Sleep Heart Health Study. Sleep 2001;24:96–105.

17. Finn L, Young T, Palta M, et al. Sleep-disordered breathing and self-reported general health status in the Wisconsin Sleep Cohort Study. Sleep 1998; 21:701–6.

18. Weiss JW, Remsburg S, Garpestad E, et al. Hemodynamic consequences of obstructive sleep apnea. Sleep 1996;19:388–97.

19. Sica AL, Greenberg HE, Ruggiero DA, et al. Chronic-intermittent hypoxia: a model of sympathetic activation in the rat. Respir Physiol 2000;121:173–84.

20. Morgan BJ, Crabtree DC, Puleo DS, et al. Neurocirculatory consequences of abrupt change in sleep state in humans. J Appl Phys 1996;80:1627–36.

21. Robinson GV, Stradling JR, Davies RJ. Sleep. 6: obstructive sleep apnoea/hypopnoea syndrome and hypertension. Thorax 2004;59:1089–94.

22. Nieto FJ, Young TB, Lind BK, et al. Association of sleep-disordered breathing, sleep apnea, and hypertension in a large community-based study. Sleep Heart Health Study. JAMA 2000;283:1829–36.

23. Hla KM, Young TB, Bidwell T, et al. Sleep apnea and hypertension. A population-based study. Ann Intern Med 1994;120:382–8.

24. Young T, Peppard P, Palta M, et al. Population-based study of sleep-disordered breathing as a risk factor for hypertension. Arch Intern Med 1997;157: 1746–52.

25. Bixler EO, Vgontzas AN, Lin HM, et al. Association of hypertension and sleep-disordered breathing. Arch Intern Med 2000;160:2289–95.

26. Peppard PE, Young T, Palta M, et al. Prospective study of the association between sleep-disordered breathing and hypertension. N Engl J Med 2000; 342:1378–84.

27. Shahar E, Whitney CW, Redline S, et al. Sleep-disordered breathing and cardiovascular disease: cross-sectional results of the Sleep Heart Health Study. Am J Respir Crit Care Med 2001;163:19–25.

28. Marin JM, Carrizo SJ, Vicente E, et al. Long-term cardiovascular outcomes in men with obstructive sleep apnoea-hypopnoea with or without treatment with continuous positive airway pressure: an observational study. Lancet 2005;365:1046–53.

29. Punjabi NM, Ahmed MM, Polotsky VY, et al. Sleep-disordered breathing, glucose intolerance, and insulin resistance. Respir Physiolo Neurobiol 2003; 136:167–78.

30. Tasali E, Mokhlesi B, Van CE. Obstructive sleep apnea and type 2 diabetes: interacting epidemics. Chest 2008;133:496–506.

31. Punjabi NM, Shahar E, Redline S, et al. Sleep-disordered breathing, glucose intolerance, and insulin resistance: the Sleep Heart Health Study. Am J Epidemiol 2004;160:521–30.

32. Ayas NT, White DP, Al-Delaimy WK, et al. A prospective study of self-reported sleep duration and incident diabetes in women. Diabetes Care 2003;26:380–4.

33. Spiegel K, Leproult R, Van CE. Impact of sleep debt on metabolic and endocrine function. Lancet 1999; 354:1435–9.

34. Kato M, Phillips BG, Sigurdsson G, et al. Effects of sleep deprivation on neural circulatory control. Hypertension 2000;35:1173–5.

35. Meier-Ewert HK, Ridker PM, Rifai N, et al. Effect of sleep loss on C-reactive protein, an inflammatory marker of cardiovascular risk. J Am Coll Cardiol 2004;43:678–83.

Epidemiology of Age-Dependence in Sleep-Disordered Breathing in Old Age: The Bay Area Sleep Cohort

Donald L. Bliwise, PhD

KEYWORDS

- Aging • Sleep apnea • Sleep disordered breathing
- Spirometry • Body mass index

Age dependence refers to a physiologic vulnerability whose likelihood increases with chronologic age.[1] Sleep disordered breathing (SDB) has been proposed as a condition whose prevalence at least partially reflects such age dependence.[2–4] During middle age, SDB is thought to represent an age-related phenomenon conferring a distinct window of vulnerability (**Fig. 1**)[2] in association with various morbidities. Indeed, Several analyses from the Sleep Heart Health Study (SHHS) have suggested that cardiovascular outcomes of SDB, such as hypertension, stroke, endothelial dysfunction, and myocardial infarct, may be more likely to occur in middle-aged, rather than older populations,[5–9] although data from other elderly cohorts[10,11] (who may be less subject to survivor bias by virtue of enrolling subjects either at a younger age or by not excluding elderly individuals who may be unusually healthy) often do not concur.

A key feature of age dependence is that effects of advancing age are assumed broadly to operate in concert with other physiologic systems undergoing aging.[12,13] Sehl and Yates[14] have articulated and refined this biomarker concept further by examining rates of change (typically as yearly percentage change in function in the measurement of a particular marker) across various organ systems, including measurements of endocrine, musculoskeletal, autonomic, and cardiovascular function. Because SDB is multidetermined, age-dependent changes in such systems could be important for understanding risk factors for the condition (**Fig. 2**).[15] Of particular interest when discussing SDB and aging are age-dependent declines in pulmonary function, most typically indexed as changes in forced vital capacity (FVC) and forced expiratory volume in 1 second (FEV_1). Age-dependent change in FVC and FEV_1 have been documented and consist of change of about 25 to 40 mL/y based on cross-sectional data.[16–18] Whether such changes have any bearing upon SDB in old age remain unexplored.

INTRODUCTION TO THE BAY AREA SLEEP COHORT

The existence of a previously established, prospectively studied cohort (Bay Area Sleep Cohort, BASC), which has been described in greater detail previously,[10,19–21] has allowed some understanding of age dependence in SDB using longitudinal data. Most knowledge about SDB in adulthood and old age derives from

This article was supported by the following grants: AG-020269, AG-06066, and AG-02504.
Program in Sleep, Aging and Chronobiology, Emory University School of Medicine, Wesley Woods Health Center, 1841 Clifton Road, Room 509, Atlanta, GA 30329, USA
E-mail address: dbliwis@emory.edu

Sleep Med Clin 4 (2009) 57–64
doi:10.1016/j.jsmc.2008.11.004
1556-407X/08/$ – see front matter

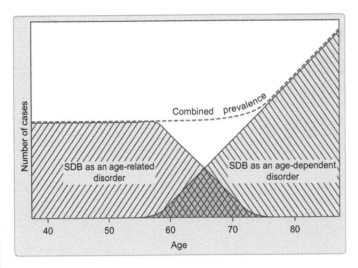

Fig. 1. Heuristic model suggesting sleep disordered breathing (SDB) as an age-dependent condition in elderly persons, relative to SDB as an age-related condition, primarily affecting middle-aged adults. Note that such a model predicts incident cases of SDB in old age should increase with advancing years (see age results in **Table 4**). (*From* Bliwise DL. Normal aging. In: Kryger MH, Roth T, Dement WC, editors. Principles and practice of sleep medicine. Philadelphia: Saunders/Elsevier; 2005. p. 33; with permission.)

cross-sectional studies. The goals in the current analyses of BASC were: to document whether SDB increases over time within individuals and determine the rate of those changes, and to examine relationships between two candidate biomarkers of age dependence, SDB and lung volumes, when both are studied over time. It was hypothesized that steeper rates of decline in FVC and FEV_1 would be associated with steeper rates of increases in SDB.

BASC originated as a convenience sample of independently living middle-aged and elderly subjects (primarily Caucasian) residing in the mid-peninsula region south of San Francisco recruited between 1974 and 1985. All participants gave informed consent, and the study was approved by the institutional review board. Individuals who had serious health problems (history of cancer, myocardial infarct, stroke, cardiac surgery, neurodegenerative diseases) were excluded from the cohort at entry. Individuals who had controlled medical conditions (eg, hypertension, arthritis) were allowed. All subjects in this report remained healthy throughout the observation period and were free from neurodegenerative diseases (eg,

dementia) or congestive heart failure at time of follow-up. BASC represented a population somewhat overselected for insomnia at entry, as many subjects subsequently were enrolled in pharmacologic trials. More completion descriptions of the original 256 members of the cohort are provided in previous publications.[10,21] None of these individuals underwent treatment of SDB during the window of observation presented here.

The subjects presented here are 103 individuals whose sleep was studied polysomnographically on two separate occasions (hereafter labeled Time 1 and Time 2) a minimum of 60 months apart (mean = 82.2 months, SD = 12.5, range 60 to 121). **Table 1** compares baseline characteristics at time of entry for the 103 participants in this follow-up from the 153 individuals not participating in this follow-up and indicates that individuals reported on here were less likely to have self-reported poor sleep but were otherwise comparable in terms of demographics and comorbid cardiovascular and psychiatric comorbidity, as indexed by medication usage. Mean age of the 103 participants at Time 1 was 66.2 (±8.2) and consisted of 34 men and 69 women; men were

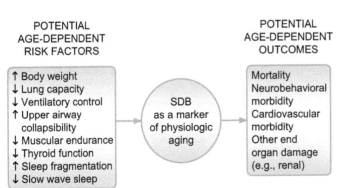

POTENTIAL AGE-DEPENDENT RISK FACTORS		POTENTIAL AGE-DEPENDENT OUTCOMES
↑ Body weight ↓ Lung capacity ↓ Ventilatory control ↑ Upper airway collapsibility ↓ Muscular endurance ↓ Thyroid function ↑ Sleep fragmentation ↓ Slow wave sleep	SDB as a marker of physiologic aging	Mortality Neurobehavioral morbidity Cardiovascular morbidity Other end organ damage (e.g., renal)

Fig. 2. Potential age-dependent risk factors and outcomes of sleep disordered breathing in old age. (*From* Bliwise DL. Normal aging. In: Kryger MH, Roth T, Dement WC, editors. Principles and practice of sleep medicine. Philadelphia: Saunders/Elsevier; 2005. p. 34; with permission.)

Table 1
Comparison of baseline (entry) data from subjects included and subjects not included in current analyses

Variable	Included (n = 103)	Not included (n = 153)	Comparison
X (SD) age (at entry) (years)	64.7 (8.7)	65.5 (9.6)	t = .69, P = .49
% Male	33.0	32.0	χ^2 = .03, P = .87
Percent with insomnia	44.7	66.7	χ^2 = 12.22, P = .0005
Percent receiving CV Rx	16.5	24.8	χ^2 = 2.53, P = .11
Percent receiving psychoactive Rx	14.6	19.0	χ^2 = .83, P = .36
X (SD) BMI (kg/m^2)	24.1 (3.6)	25.0 (4.0)	t = 1.62, P = .11
X (SD) TST (PSG) (minutes)	362.2 (84.9)	358.0 (93.2)	t = .36, P = .72
X (SD) SE (PSG) (%)	74.5 (14.8)	73.2 (15.8)	t = .70, P = .48
X (SD) PLMSI (events/hour)	14.2 (23.8)	19.7 (28.5)	t = 1.52, P = .13
X (SD) typical sleep duration (minutes) (self-report)	407.8 (74.2)	373.8 (86.7)	t = 3.10, P = .002

Abbreviations: BMI, body mass index; CV Rx, cardiovascular medication, includes hydrochlorothiazide, beta blockers, alpha blockers, calcium-channel blockers, angiotensin-converting enzyme inhibitors, lipid-lowering agents, nitrates, diuretics, and cardiac arrhythmia medications including those containing digitalis; PLMSI, periodic leg movements in sleep per sleep hour; psychoactive Rx, psychoactive medication, includes anxiolytics, sedative/hypnotics, antidepressants, neuroleptics; SE, sleep efficiency; TST, total sleep time.

significantly older than women (68.9 [±8.3] versus 64.9 [±8.0], t = 2.38, P = .019).

All 103 individuals underwent in-laboratory polysomnography (PSG), height and weight measurements, and pulmonary function tests (PFTs) at Time 1 and Time 2 evaluations. Most participants (58 at Time 1, 98 at Time 2) had two more nights of polysomnography, and in those cases, nights were averaged within subjects. For those subjects who had only one night of recording (45 at Time 1, 5 at Time 2), data from that single night were used in all subsequent calculations.

Because concurrent use of spirometry was not always available at baseline, the Time 1 measurements here represent data during the 1974 to 1985 entry window for only a subset of the 103 participants (n = 62). For the remaining 41 cases, the Time 1 data presented here represent polysomnographic, spirometric, and body weight data collected at a date subsequent to entry into BASC, but at least 60 months apart from the Time 2 measurement. All Time 2 data were derived from the 1987 to 1992 round of follow-up.

Polysomnography

PSG was performed with Grass Model 78 polysomnographs (Grass Instruments, Quincy, Massachusetts) and scored on paper by trained technologists not familiar with the body weight or spirometry data of the participants. Details of the montage can be found elsewhere.[10] Breathing

disturbance in sleep was quantified as the apnea/hypopnea index (AHI), with apneas classified by a complete cessation of breathing and hypopneas classified by a reduction in airflow of at least 50% from the immediately preceding baseline. For the analyses described here a minimal desaturation criterion or an arousal criterion were not used to qualify hypopneas. Previous analyses from this cohort showed a similar pattern of results in association with outcomes regardless of hypopnea definition.[10] AHI as a summed metric retains high inter-rater reliability within the laboratory's recording and scoring procedures.[22] Most events (74%) were scored as obstructive/mixed rather than central. All scoring was performed blind to patients' spirometry results.

Body Mass Index

Heights (m) and weights (kg) were derived from a standard clinic scale with participants fully clothed but with shoes removed. Body mass index (BMI) was calculated as weight/height.^{2}

Spirometry

Spirometry was performed at Time 1 and Time 2 for all BASC subjects included in the current report. Standard maneuvers followed American Thoracic Society Snowbird Workshop guidelines for measurements of FVC and FEV$_1$, employing the best of three trials.[23] Studies were done in standing position using nose clips. Following the procedures of Knudson and colleagues,[24] each subject's highest FVC and FEV$_1$ were used, even if they were derived from two different maneuvers.[25]

At Time 1, spirometry was performed with a portable bellows unit (Waters Spirometer, Model Pulmonarie 10, Jones, Oakbrook, Illinois), which was checked regularly with a 3 L calibration syringe. Time 2 testing was performed in the Stanford University Medical Center Pulmonary Function Laboratory using a water-based volume displacement spirometer (Collins DS system, Warren Collins, Braintree, Massachusetts). To adjust for possible effects of use of different equipment at Time 1 and Time 2, 65 of the 103 participants at Time 2 were retested with the portable spirometer the same day as the in-hospital measurements were made. Linear regression demonstrated an extremely high concordance between the portable and in-laboratory measurements (for FVC, r^2 = .928, F=700.22, P<.0001, slope = 1.10, intercept = .208; for FEV$_1$, r^2 = .933, F = 882.91, P<.0001, slope = 1.08, intercept = .110) and suggested that the portable unit slightly, but consistently, underestimated volumes. To correct for this small underestimation of FVC and FEV$_1$ on Time 1 measurements, all Time 1 spirometric measurements were adjusted to correct for these differences (for FVC, portable FVC × 1.10 + .208; for FEV$_1$, portable FEV$_1$ × 1.08 + .111).

FINDINGS FROM THE CURRENT ANALYSES OF THE BAY AREA SLEEP COHORT

Table 2 shows Time 1 and Time 2 data on BASC subjects; simple t-tests suggested that AHI increased over time for men and women. For all time-dependent measures (ie, AHI, BMI, FVC, and FEV$_1$), rates of change, calculated as the

Table 2
Change in time-dependent variables

	Time 1	Time 2	Change
Variable			
Apnea/hypopnea index (AHI) (events/h)			
Women	1.95 (2.77)	4.51 (6.67)	t = 3.86, P = .0003
Men	9.69 (11.30)	16.11 (17.40)	t = 3.40, P = .0018
Both	4.51 (7.74)	8.34 (12.56)	t = 4.91, P < .0001
LogAHI			
Women	.79 (.70)	1.34 (.78)	t = 6.53, P < .0001
Men	1.88 (1.03)	2.34 (1.04)	t = 4.09, P = .0003
Both	1.15 (.96)	1.67 (.99)	t = 7.72, P < .0001
Weight (kg)			
Women	64.24 (12.20)	65.52 (14.13)	t = 1.62, P = .109
Men	75.15 (11.60)	74.35 (12.87)	t = .79, P = .433
Both	67.84 (13.01)	68.44 (14.28)	t = .94, P = .35
Body mass index (kg/m^2)			
Women	24.01 (4.04)	24.51 (4.92)	t = 1.69, P = .096
Men	24.18 (2.51)	23.90 (2.98)	t = .87, P = .39
Both	24.07 (3.59)	24.31 (4.37)	t = 1.05, P = .30
Forced vital capacity (L)			
Women	2.79 (.66)	2.50 (.65)	t = 6.33, P < .0001
Men	3.93 (.84)	3.64 (.84)	t = 2.77, P = .009
Both	3.17 (.90)	2.88 (.90)	t = 6.30, P < .0001
Forced expiratory volume in 1 s (L)			
Women	2.05 (.57)	1.88 (.55)	t = 4.54, P < .0001
Men	2.77 (.62)	2.57 (.68)	t = 1.76, P = .087
Both	2.29 (.67)	2.11 (.68)	t = 4.04, P < .0001

Data presented as X (SD).

Time 2 value of each measurement minus the Time 1 value of each measurement divided by number of months of follow-up, were computed. These rates then were multiplied by 12 to derive a rate of change per year. AHI data are presented as both raw and log transformed (calculated as log[1 + AHI] to correct for skew) values (**Table 2**), although only the latter were used for correlational analyses.

Rates of change in AHI over time are shown in **Table 3** for men and women and suggest slightly higher rates of change for men. Overall, the median rate of change in AHI was .188 events/h/y (range: −2.50 to +5.69), with 81 cases showing increases, 20 cases showing decreases, and 2 without change. These data indicated that BASC members were far more likely to increase, rather than decrease, their AHI over time.

With regards to body weight, BASC women gained (within subjects analyses) on average 1.28 kg (SD=6.53), whereas men lost -.80 kg (SD 5.86) over the years of observation (mean group values shown on **Table 2**). These changes were not statistically significant. Rates of change in FVC and FEV_1 averaged 47 and 32 mL/y for men, respectively, and 40 and 24 mL/y for women, respectively (**Table 3**), approximating rates of change in these measures in previously published normative data.[16–18]

Table 4 shows data relevant to age dependence in AHI. Over the 7 years of observation, steeper rates of decline in yearly rates for FVC and FEV_1 were related to increased rates in AHI, those relationships somewhat more pronounced for men than for women. These data suggest a critical association between these two biomarkers (SDB and lung volumes) within BASC. Yearly rates of change in AHI were related marginally to older age at entry in men but not in women.

IMPLICATIONS OF THE CURRENT FINDINGS: SPIROMETRY AND AGE DEPENDENCE IN SLEEP DISORDERED BREATHING

Numerous cross-sectional studies generally have suggested little utility in traditional spirometric measures in predicting individuals who have SDB. Although initial enthusiasm for the determination of sleep-related upper airway obstruction from measures such as flow volume loops was high,[26] most measures derived from routine PFTs were considered to hold little prognostic value in sleep clinic patients.[27] Studies examining the pathophysiology of SDB in old age instead have focused on age-dependent changes in upper airway structure or function.[28–31] Placed in this context, the current results suggesting that declining FVC and FEV_1 may be associated with incident SDB over time may appear surprising.

More careful consideration of the complex interactive effects between upper and lower airway function in SDB, however, yields a potential basis for such an effect. Cross-sectional area in the upper airway long has been known to be dependent upon lung volumes,[32–36] and experimental evidence has shown that increased functional residual capacity (by experimentally applied negative extrathoracic pressures) reduces SDB.[33] Recent mechanistic studies examining muscle activity and upper airway collapsibility in normal subjects subjected to manipulations in extrathoracic pressure have confirmed that as lung volumes increased, collapsibility decreased, although the role of altered genioglossus activity appears unlikely to be the basis of the effect.[37] A more likely explanation involves the mechanism sometimes referred to as the tracheal tug, which has been modeled in dogs[38] and is thought to represent the caudal displacement of the trachea, resulting

Table 3
Gender differences in yearly rate of change

Variable	Women (n = 69)	Men (n = 34)	Combined (n = 103)	Comparison
Body mass index (kg/m²/year)	.064 (.331)	−.046 (.332)	.027 (.333)	t = 1.58, P = .12
Forced vital capacity (L/year)	−.040 (.053)	−.047 (.103)	−.043 (.073)	t = .33, P = .74
Forced expiratory volume in 1 s (L/y)	−.024 (.044)	−.032 (.106)	−.027 (.070)	t = .40, P = .69
Apnea/hypopnea index (AHI) (events/h/y)	.36 (.82)	1.10 (1.94)	.61 (1.33)	t = 2.12, P = .04
LogAHI (events/h/y)	.076 (.100)	.076 (.109)	.076 (.103)	t=0.0, P = .99

Values in first three columns represent X (SD) of change rate (in units shown); final column shows two-group *t*-tests for gender comparisons.

Table 4
Correlations between yearly log transformed rate of change in apnea/hypopnea index and key variables

Variable	Women (n=69)	Men (n=34)	Combined (n=103)
Time 1 age	.139 (.254)	.324 (.062)	.199 (.044)
Body mass index yearly change (kg/m²/y)	−.052 (.669)	−.206 (.242)	−.104 (.295)
Forced vital capacity yearly change (L/y)	−.114 (.351)	−.414 (.015)	−.187 (.059)
Forced expiratory volume in 1 s yearly change (L/y)	−.214 (.078)	−.208 (.238)	−.183 (.064)

Pearson correlations shown; *p* values in parentheses.

in stiffening of the upper airway musculature from mechanical forces. These findings suggest that the development of SDB in older adults might derive at least partially from such mechanical factors (eg, declines in chest wall compliance and loss of elastic recoil)[39] that could manifest in steeper rates of decline in FVC and FEV_1. In this regard, it may be informative to re-examine the largely negative findings of relationships between routine pulmonary function measures and SDB. For example, one large case series of PSG and PFT data in sleep apnea indicated that FVC and FEV_1 decreased with increased severity of SDB.[40] Those effects disappeared when age was controlled, however, and the effects were interpreted largely as indicating that lung volumes were of minimal significance in the prediction of SDB. Data such as these are compatible with the longitudinal data presented here, in which age was a time-dependent covariate (by definition), and the passage of time (aging) was associated with lung-volume dependent increases in SDB. The data are also consistent with reports from a small cohort of healthy older individuals, for whom elevated baseline AHI measurements (AHI greater than 5) showed persistent relationship to reduced pulmonary function.[41,42]

Body weight changes were not noted in relation to incident SDB in BASC. In cross-sectional analyses from the SHHS,[43] elevated BMI was noted to confer a decreased magnitude of risk for SDB in older age groups, and a similarly reduced role of changes in BMI for incident SDB was noted in SHHS longitudinal data over a 5-year interval.[44] In longitudinal population-based data encompassing younger subjects, the Wisconsin Sleep Cohort Study (WSCS)[45] and the Cleveland Family Study (CFS)[46,47] noted that increases and decreases in body weight over time were associated with increases and decreases in AHI, respectively, although in CFS, the magnitude of body weight effects were tempered among older cohort members.[46] Regardless of differential strength of associations with body weight changes, all of these studies uniformly reported increases in AHI over time, which is consistent with what has been noted in BASC. Some previous longitudinal studies of sleep in older adults did not find increased SDB over time,[48,49] but did not rely on laboratory-based polysomnography and used smaller samples than are reported here. In contrast to all of these previous studies, BASC affords a somewhat unique perspective on the SDB of old age by virtue of simultaneous PFT measurements and repeated nights of PSG.

What are the implications of a possible impact of lung volumes in the prediction of long-term development of SDB or even its prevention? Maintenance of healthy pulmonary function throughout the human life span long has been recognized to be related to avoidance of aversive environmental exposures, avoidance of smoking, and appropriate nutrition in the presence of ideal body weight. Salutary influences on lung function, such as exercise, may have beneficial effects on SDB that do not depend on body weight.[50–52] To the extent that lung volumes predict development of SDB over time, maintenance of healthy aerobic capacity might be protective to some extent for development of SDB in old age.

SUMMARY

SDB is highly prevalent in elderly populations and is thought to reflect, at least in part, age dependence. Several studies suggest that SDB in elderly populations may hold different functional outcomes relative to SDB in middle-aged populations. Risk factors for SDB specific for the elderly remain uncertain. This article examined changes in SDB, body weight, and pulmonary function in 103 individuals over an average interval of 7 years to determine whether changes in these measures covaried. In-laboratory PSG was performed on members of an elderly cohort (BASC) on two separate occasions (Time 1, Time 2), with multiple nights of measurement typically made on each occasion. Results indicated that:

- SDB progressed over time in men and women
- Changes in body weight were unrelated to the progression in SDB
- Relative declines in lung volumes (FVC, FEV_1) were associated with relative increases in SDB, with the effects slightly stronger in men

These data suggest that age dependence in one commonly ascribed aging biomarker (lung function) was coupled with increments in SDB. Maintenance of healthy lung function into old age may confer some protective benefits in the development of age-dependent SDB.

ACKNOWLEDGMENTS

I gratefully acknowledge the following individuals for their invaluable assistance in collecting and analyzing data on Bay Area Sleep Cohort: Farzaneh Pour Ansari, Sophia A. Greer, Ann Pursley Kollrack, Julia Zarcone Pattmore, Laura-Beth Straight, and the Pulmonary Function Laboratory at Stanford University Medical School.

REFERENCES

1. Brody JA, Schneider EL. Diseases and disorders of aging: an hypothesis. J Chronic Dis 1986;39:871–6.
2. Young T. Age dependence of sleep disordered breathing. In: Kuna ST, Suratt PM, Remmers JE, editors. Sleep and respiration in aging adults. New York: Elsevier; 1991. p. 161–70.
3. Bliwise DL. Sleep in normal aging and dementia. Sleep 1993;16:40–81.
4. Bliwise DL. Chronological age, physiological age, and mortality in sleep apnea [editorial]. Sleep 1996;19:275–6.
5. Haas DC, Foster GL, Nieto FJ, et al. Age-dependent associations between sleep-disordered breathing and hypertension: importance of discriminating between systolic/diastolic hypertension and isolated systolic hypertension in the Sleep Heart Health Study. Circulation 2005;111:614–25.
6. Nieto FJ, Young TB, Lind BK, et al. Association of sleep-disordered breathing, sleep apnea, and hypertension in a large community-based study. JAMA 2000;283:1829–36.
7. Nieto FJ, Herrington DM, Redline S, et al. Sleep apnea and markers of vascular endothelial function in a large community sample of older adults. Am J Respir Crit Care Med 2004;169:354–60.
8. Newman AB, Nieto FJ, Guidry U, et al. Relation of sleep-disordered breathing to cardiovascular disease risk factors: the Sleep Heart Health Study. Am J Epidemiol 2001;154:50–9.
9. Shahar E, Whitney CW, Redline S, et al. Sleep-disordered breathing and cardiovascular disease: cross-sectional results of the Sleep Heart Health Study. Am J Respir Crit Care Med 2001;163:19–25.
10. Endeshaw YW, Bloom HL, Bliwise DL. Sleep-disordered breathing and cardiovascular disease in the Bay Area Sleep Cohort. Sleep 2008;31:563–8.
11. Mehra R, Stone KL, Blackwell T, et al. Prevalence and correlates of sleep-disordered breathing in older men: osteoporotic fractures in men sleep study. J Am Geriatr Soc 2007;55:1356–64.
12. Dement WC, Miles LE, Bliwise DL. Physiological markers of aging: human sleep pattern changes. Publication #NIH 82-2221. In: Reff ME, Schneider EL, editors. Biological markers of aging. Washington, DC: US Department of Health and Human Services; 1982. p. 177–87.
13. Kannel WB, Hubert H. Vital capacity as a biomarker of aging. Publication #NIH 82-2221. In: Reff ME, Schneider EL, editors. Biological markers of aging. Washington, DC: U.S. Department of Health and Human Service; 1982. p. 145–60.
14. Sehl ME, Yates FE. Kinetics of human aging: I. rates of senescence between ages 30 and 70 years in healthy people. J Gerontol A Biol Sci Med Sci 2001;56A:B198–208.
15. Bliwise DL. Normal aging. In: Kryger MH, Roth T, Dement WC, editors. Principles and practice of sleep medicine. 4th edition. Philadelphia: Saunders/Elsevier; 2005. p. 24–38.
16. Morris JF, Koski A, Johnson LC. Spirometric standards for healthy nonsmoking adults. Am Rev Respir Dis 1971;103:57–67.
17. Dhar S, Shastri SR, Lenora RAK. Aging and the respiratory system. Med Clin North Am 1976;60:1121–39.
18. Smith WDF, Cunningham DA, Patterson DH, et al. Forced expiratory volume, height and demispan in Canadian men and women aged 55–86. J Gerontol A Biol Sci Med Sci 1992;47:M40–4.
19. Bliwise DL, Bliwise NG, Partinen M, et al. Sleep apnea and mortality in an aged cohort. Am J Public Health 1988;78:544–7.
20. Bliwise DL, Feldman DE, Bliwise NG, et al. Risk factors for sleep disordered breathing in heterogeneous geriatric populations. J Am Geriatr Soc 1987;35:132–41.
21. Bliwise DL. Sleep and aging. In: Pressman MR, Orr WC, editors. Understanding sleep: the evaluation and treatment of sleep disorders. Washington, DC: American Psychological Association; 1997. p. 441–64.
22. Bliwise D, Bliwise NG, Kraemer HC, et al. Measurement error in visually scored electrophysiological

data: respiration during sleep. J Neurosci Methods 1984;12:49–56.

23. American Thoracic Society. ATS statement—Snowbird Workshop on standardization of spirometry. Am Rev Respir Dis 1979;119:831–8.

24. Knudson RJ, Lebowitz MD, Holberg CJ, et al. Changes in the normal maximal expiratory flow volume curve with growth and aging. Am Rev Respir Dis 1983;127:725–34.

25. American Thoracic Society. Standardization of spirometry—1987 update. Am Rev Respir Dis 1987;136:1285–98.

26. Sanders MH, Martin RJ, Pennock BE, et al. The detection of sleep apnea in the awake patient: the sawtooth sign. JAMA 1981;243:2414–8.

27. Katz I, Zamel N, Slutsky AS, et al. An evaluation of flow volume curves as a screening test for obstructive sleep apnea. Chest 1990;98:337–40.

28. Brown IG, Zamel N, Hoffstein V. Pharyngeal cross-sectional area in normal men and women. J Appl Phys 1986;61:890–5.

29. Martin SE, Marthur R, Marshall I, et al. The effects of age, sex, obesity, and posture on upper airway size. Eur Respir J 1997;10:2087–90.

30. McGinty D, Littner M, Beahm E, et al. Sleep-related breathing disorders in older men: a search for underlying mechanisms. Neurobiol Aging 1982;3:337–50.

31. White DF, Lombard RM, Cadieux RJ, et al. Pharyngeal resistance in normal humans: influence of gender, age and obesity. J Appl Phys 1985;58:365–71.

32. Brooks LJ, Byard PJ, Helms RC, et al. Relationship between lung volume and tracheal area as assessed by acoustic reflection. J Appl Phys 1988;64:1050–4.

33. Series F, Cormier Y, Lampron N, et al. Influence of lung volume in sleep apnoea. Thorax 1989;44:52–7.

34. Series F, Cormier Y, Desmeules M. Influence of passive changes of lung volume on upper airways. J Appl Phys 1990;68:2159–64.

35. Series F, Marc I. Influence of lung volume dependence of upper airway resistance during continuous negative airway pressure. J Appl Phys 1994;77:840–4.

36. Stauffer JL, White DP, Zwillich CW. Pulmonary function in obstructive sleep apnea: relationships to pharyngeal resistance and cross-sectional area. Chest 1990;97:302–7.

37. Stanchina ML, Malhotra A, Fogel RB, et al. The influence of lung volume on pharyngeal mechanics, collapsibility, and genioglossus muscle activation during sleep. Sleep 2003;26:851–6.

38. Van de Graaff WB. Thoracic influence on upper airway patency. J Appl Phys 1988;65:2124–31.

39. Pack AI, Millman RP. Changes in control of ventilation, awake and asleep, in the elderly. J Am Geriatr Soc 1986;34:533–44.

40. Hoffstein V, Oliver Z. Pulmonary function and sleep apnea. Sleep Breath 2003;7:159–65.

41. Phillips BA, Berry DT, Lipke-Molby TC. Sleep-disordered breathing in healthy, aged persons. Fifth and final year follow-up. Chest 1996;110:654–8.

42. Phillips BA, Berry DTR, Schmitt FA, et al. Sleep disordered breathing in healthy aged persons: two- and three-year follow-up. Sleep 1994;17:411–5.

43. Young T, Shahar E, Nieto FJ, et al. Predictors of sleep-disordered breathing in community-dwelling adults: the Sleep Heart Health Study. Arch Intern Med 2002;162:893–900.

44. Newman AB, Foster G, Givelber R, et al. Progression and regression of sleep-disordered breathing with changes in weight. Arch Intern Med 2005;165:2408–13.

45. Peppard PE, Young T, Palta M, et al. Longitudinal study of moderate weight change and sleep-disordered breathing. JAMA 2000;284:3015–21.

46. Redline S, Schluchter MD, Larkin EK, et al. Predictors of longitudinal change in sleep-disordered breathing in a nonclinic population. Sleep 2003;26:703–9.

47. Tishler PV, Larkin EK, Schluchter MD, et al. Incidence of sleep-disordered breathing in an urban adult population; the relative importance of risk factors in the development of sleep-disordered breathing. JAMA 2003;289:2230–7.

48. Ancoli-Israel S, Kripke DF, Klauber MR, et al. Natural history of sleep disordered breathing in community dwelling elderly. Sleep 1993;16:S25–9.

49. Ancoli-Israel S, Gehrman P, Kripke DF, et al. Long-term follow-up of sleep disordered breathing in older adults. Sleep Med 2001;2:511–6.

50. Giebelhaus V, Strohl KP, Lormes W, et al. Physical exercise as an adjunct therapy in sleep apnea—an open trial. Sleep Breath 2000;4:173–6.

51. Norman JF, Von Essen SG, Fuchs RH, et al. Exercise training effect on obstructive sleep apnea syndrome. Sleep Res Online 2000;3:121–9.

52. Peppard PE, Young T. Exercise and sleep disordered breathing: an association independent of body habitus. Sleep 2004;27:480–4.

Obesity and Self-Reported Short Sleep Duration: A Marker of Sleep Complaints and Chronic Psychosocial Stress

Alexandros N. Vgontzas, MD*, Slobodanka Pejovic, MD, Susan Calhoun, PhD, Edward O. Bixler, PhD

KEYWORDS

- Obesity • Self-reported short sleep duration
- Sleep complaints • Stress • Objective sleep duration
- Cardiometabolic morbidity

Obesity is highly prevalent in the modern world. In the United States the prevalence of obesity has increased significantly over the past two decades. In 1980, 15% of American adults were obese with a body mass index (BMI) greater than or equal to 30, whereas in 2000, the number doubled to 30.4% (with 33.2% women and 27.6% men affected).[1]

In addition to the well-established role of conditions such as diet, nutrition, and exercise, chronic sleep restriction has been recently identified as a novel factor that may explain the increasing prevalence of obesity.[2] Several surveys have shown that American adults currently sleep significantly less than in the beginning of the twentieth century.[3,4] In addition, many studies have demonstrated that increased levels of obesity are associated with decreased sleep duration.[5–11] Furthermore, a number of physiologic studies have shown that experimentally induced, short-term sleep deprivation may predispose healthy individuals to weight gain by increasing appetite, and thus caloric intake, as a result of altered levels of appetite-regulating peptides, such as leptin and ghrelin.[12,13] This evidence combined has led to the widely held position that sleep curtailment is a novel risk factor for weight gain and obesity.

Most of the epidemiologic studies reporting on the association of short sleep duration and obesity are based on self-reports, whereas studies using objective sleep measures are limited and have reported either a weak or no association between the two. In the sleep field, the association between self-reported and objective measures of sleep has been modest, and the interpretation of this phenomenon has been a challenge. In particular, for some types of patients, such as insomniacs, self-reported sleep is typically an underestimate of their true objective sleep. More recently, it has been shown that, in general population samples also, the correlation between self-reported and objective measures of sleep are modest and, in contrast to clinical samples, subjective reports are based on systematic overreporting.[14]

The discrepancy between self-reported versus measured sleep raises a significant scientific and clinical question: what is subjective sleep duration associated with? What are the clinical profiles and characteristics of obese individuals who report short sleep? Does the self-reported sleep duration

Department of Psychiatry, Sleep Research and Treatment Center, Penn State College of Medicine, H073, 500 University Drive, Hershey, PA 17033, USA
* Corresponding author.
E-mail address: avgontzas@hmc.psu.edu (A.N. Vgontzas).

Sleep Med Clin 4 (2009) 65–75
doi:10.1016/j.jsmc.2009.01.001

reflect voluntary sleep restriction, sleep complaints, or increased psychosocial stress?

In the first part of this article, we address these questions using data from the large Penn State cohort in adults.[15] Next, we present a critical review of the few studies that used objective measures of sleep and how these findings can be understood in view of the findings from subjective studies. Finally, we provide a unified hypothesis of how short sleep duration, both subjective or objective, is useful in evaluating and treating obese individuals.

PENN STATE COHORT: SHORT SLEEP DURATION AND OBESITY

In this study, 741 men and 1000 women were randomly selected from the general population in central Pennsylvania, and each subject was studied in our sleep laboratory.[15] They completed a comprehensive medical evaluation, including sleep history and physical examination, and the Minnesota Multiphasic Personality Inventory-2 (MMPI-2).[16] BMI was based on height and weight measured as part of the physical examination. Thirteen hundred (1300) completed a valid MMPI-2. For the purposes of this study, sleep apnea was defined as an obstructive apnea or hypopnea index (OHI) 15 or greater (OHI $\geq$ 15). Also, objective sleep duration was based on percentage sleep time (%ST). In addition, for those subjects who participated in the polysomnographic phase of this study, we subjectively assessed, "how many hours do you usually sleep at night?"

We further assessed for the presence of all sleep disorders. The presence of insomnia was established on two levels of severity.[17] First, insomnia was defined by a complaint of insomnia with a duration of at least one year. Second, difficulty sleeping was defined as a moderate to severe complaint of difficulty falling asleep, difficulty staying asleep, early final awakening, or unrefreshed. The presence of excessive daytime sleepiness (EDS) was established based on a moderate or severe rating on either of the following two questions: "do you feel drowsy or sleepy most of the day but manage to stay awake?" and "do you have any irresistible sleep attacks during the day?"[18]

The 1300 subjects who completed a valid MMPI-2 were not different from the overall sample of 1741 in terms of age, gender, BMI, or sleep complaints. Obesity was defined in two ways: (1) BMI greater than 27.8 kg/m^2 for men and 27.3 kg/m^2 for women (criteria for overweight when our sample was collected)[19] and (2) BMI greater than 30 kg/m^2, which is the current definition of obesity.[20] In the presentation of the data we have followed the current definition of obesity except otherwise indicated. The overall subjective sleep disturbance was defined as having at least one of the following complaints: EDS, insomnia, or sleep difficulty. The chronic stress level was measured by the average of the T scores of all eight clinical subscales of MMPI-2. T scores with a mean of 50 and a standard deviation of 10 are generated for the eight major clinical scales. Scores greater than or equal to 65 (1.5 SD above the mean) indicate a significant deviation from the original normal standardization pattern of responding and suggested an elevation at a clinically significant level.

We created five categories of self-reported sleep duration:

1. Less than or equal to 5 hours
2. Greater than 5, less than or equal to 6 hours
3. Greater than 6, less than or equal to 7 hours
4. Greater than 7, less than or equal to 8 hours
5. Greater than 8 hours.

To determine the shape of the relationship between BMI and self-reported sleep duration, a scale from 1 to 5 was assigned for the five sleep duration categories. Then a piecewise regression model was fitted to test whether the slopes of the sleep duration were linear before and after 7 hours of sleep after adjusting for age and gender.

Multiple regression analysis was applied to assess the individual and joint effects of MMPI-2 and BMI on the reduction of self-reported and objective sleep durations, while adjusting for age, gender, current report of smoking, and sleep disordered breathing (SDB). To compare the relative contribution of the MMPI-2 and BMI, the magnitudes of the effects of MMPI-2 and BMI were expressed in terms of one standard deviation change.

THE ASSOCIATION BETWEEN SELF-REPORTED SLEEP DURATION AND BODY MASS INDEX IS CURVILINEAR

The characteristics of the sample are presented in **Table 1**. The BMI of our sample is somewhat high because (1) we oversampled for risk factors of SDB, including obesity, and (2) the BMI of men and women from central Pennsylvania was higher compared with the national population.[18,21,22] Because there was not a significant interaction between gender and reported sleep duration, we examined the association within the entire sample. We found a significant curvilinear relationship between average nightly sleep and BMI after adjustment for age and gender.[15] The maximum BMI was associated with an average sleep

Table 1
Demographic and sleep characteristics of 1300 men and women of a general population sample from central Pennsylvania

	Men (n = 561)	Women (n = 739)
Age	50.8 ± 12.6	54.9 ± 13.6
BMI (kg/m²)	28.8 ± 4.3	32.7 ± 7.5
% Obese	33.7	61.4
Self-reported sleep		
Duration (hours)	6.5 ± 1.3	6.8 ± 1.3
% Sleep time	71.0 ± 15.6	71.0 ± 15.8
MMPI average score		
(T values)	51.2 ± 6.6	52.8 ± 8.2
% SDB	11.76	6.09
% Smoking	27.99	13.26

duration of less than five hours. Compared with the group of subjects who slept more than 6 and less than or equal to 7 hours, BMI decreased proportionally to increased sleep for those who slept less; however, BMI remained similar for those who slept more.

SLEEP COMPLAINTS ARE FREQUENT IN OBESE SUBJECTS AND ARE ASSOCIATED WITH SHORT SLEEP DURATION

Individual sleep complaints, as well as overall, were more prevalent in the obese subjects versus nonobese subjects (47.4% versus 25.5%; $P<.01$) (**Table 2**).

Both obese men and women with sleep complaints reported shorter sleep duration compared with obese subjects without sleep complaints (**Fig. 1**). The shortest sleep duration was reported by the obese insomniacs who averaged 5.9 hours, followed by obese subjects with EDS or sleep difficulty. In contrast, obese subjects without sleep complaints reported very similar sleep duration to nonobese without complaints (7.0 hours for obese and 6.9 for nonobese subjects).

In a regression analysis that included the entire sample of 1300 subjects, both BMI and presence of any sleep complaints were significant predictors of self-reported sleep duration after adjustment for SDB, smoking, gender, and age. The association between BMI and sleep duration was linear and negative. In a stratified analysis by gender (the interaction between gender and sleep complaint was significant; $P = .01$), BMI was significant only for men. Specifically in men, for an increase of one standard deviation of BMI (about 4.3 kg/m²), reported sleep duration was reduced by approximately 7 minutes, whereas in women, an increase of BMI by one standard deviation (about 7.5 kg/m²) was associated with a reduction of reported sleep by 5 minutes. Equivalently, a 10 kg/m² increase in BMI was associated with a reduction of reported sleep by 16 minutes for men and by

Table 2
Obesity and subjective sleep disturbances prevalence in a general random population sample in the United States

	Nonobese	Obese
Insomnia	6.0% (6.1%)	11.1%[b] (9.2%)
Sleep difficulty	17.3% (16.7%)	31.5%[a] (27.2%)
EDS	7.5% (7.3%)	15.6%[a] (13.0%)
Any sleep disturbance	25.5% (24.8%)	47.4%[a] (40.7%)

Parenthetical values represent obesity defined as BMI >27.8 kg/m² for men and 27.3 kg/m² for women.
[a] $P<.01$.
[b] $P<.05$.

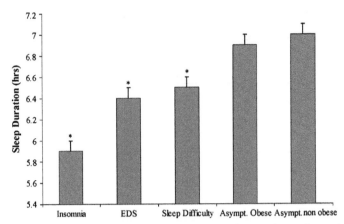

Fig. 1. Average sleep duration in obese with sleep disturbance versus obese and nonobese without subjective sleep disturbance (asymptomatic). Data represent mean values + 1 standard error. *P<.05 between obese with sleep disturbance versus obese and nonobese without sleep disturbance. (*From* Vgontzas AN, Lin HM, Papaliaga M, et al. Short sleep duration and obesity: the role of emotional stress and sleep disturbance. Int J Obes 2008;32(5):801–9; with permission.)

6 minutes for women. Furthermore, sleep complaints were significant for both genders. In men, the presence of a sleep complaint was associated with an approximately 18 minute reduction of reported sleep, whereas in women, it was associated with a reduction of sleep by 42 minutes. Notably, in men, the presence of SDB was associated with an increase of self-reported sleep duration.

Finally, we examined whether depression and medical disorders associated with physical pain/discomfort, ie, arthritis, migraine headaches, peptic ulcer/GERD, and irritable bowel syndrome were more prevalent in obese versus nonobese subjects. There was no significant difference between the two groups in terms of depression, or pain/discomfort-related physical disorders.

SELF-REPORTED SHORT SLEEP DURATION IS ASSOCIATED WITH STRESS

In a multivariate regression analysis that included the entire sample, with dependent variable self-reported sleep duration and independent variables BMI, and MMPI-2, after adjusting for age, smoking, gender, and SDB, both BMI and average MMPI-2 score were significant predictors of sleep duration. In the main effects model, the effect of MMPI-2 score was stronger than that of BMI in terms of reduction of sleep duration per one standard deviation increase of MMPI-2 or BMI, as well as of the *P* values. No significant interaction between MMPI-2 and gender was observed. However, there was a synergistic joint effect between MMPI-2 and BMI, ie, the MMPI-2 effect was modified by the BMI levels (P<.1). For an increase of MMPI-2 by

one standard deviation, the reduction of self-reported sleep was greater among the heavier subjects than in the lighter subjects. Similarly, for an increase of BMI for one standard deviation, the reduction of self-reported sleep duration was greater in the more distressed subjects than in the less distressed subjects (**Fig. 2**).

The subjects who reported sleep duration greater than 8 hours were mostly middle-aged and older subjects (75% >45 years). Interestingly, in this group of "long sleepers," sleep duration was associated with higher levels of stress (r = 0.45, P<.05) only in younger adults (age ≤45).

SELF-REPORTED SHORT SLEEP DURATION IS ASSOCIATED BOTH WITH SLEEP COMPLAINTS AND STRESS

Obese subjects with sleep complaints experienced higher levels of stress compared with those obese without sleep complaints. Specifically, obese men and women with insomnia or sleep difficulty showed significantly higher scores on all eight clinical scales of the MMPI-2 compared with those without sleep complaints (**Fig. 3**). The same pattern was noted for obese subjects with EDS versus asymptomatic (without sleep complaints) obese subjects (**Fig. 4**). However, the differences were stronger in women who reported EDS compared with men. In contrast, there was no difference in MMPI-2 profiles between asymptomatic (no sleep disturbance) nonobese versus asymptomatic obese subjects (**Fig. 5**).

In a regression analysis that included BMI, MMPI-2, and sleep complaints as independent variables, BMI was a significant predictor of self-

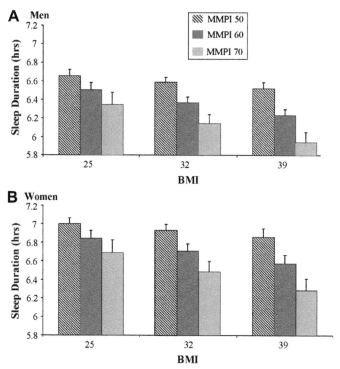

Fig. 2. Interaction of emotional stress and BMI with self-reported sleep duration. Top panel (*A*) depicts sleep duration in 50-year-old men by varying degree of obesity and stress after adjustment for age, sleep disordered breathing, and smoking. Bottom panel (*B*) illustrates the same interaction in 50-year-old women. (*From* Vgontzas AN, Lin HM, Papaliaga M, et al. Short sleep duration and obesity: the role of emotional stress and sleep disturbance. Int J Obes 2008;32(5):801–9; with permission.)

reported sleep duration after adjusting for age, smoking, gender, and SDB. The association between BMI and sleep duration was linear and negative. There was also a synergistic effect between MMPI-2 and sleep complaints. Specifically, for every unit increase of MMPI-2, the reduction of self-reported sleep was greater among those who had sleep complaints. Similarly, the

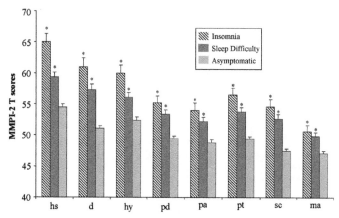

Fig. 3. MMPI profiles in asymptomatic (without sleep disturbance) obese versus obese with insomnia and sleep difficulty. Mean MMPI-2T scores + 1 standard error in all eight clinical scales after adjustment for age and gender. *P <0.05 obese with insomnia or sleep difficulty versus obese with no subjective sleep disturbance. hs, hypochondriasis; d, depression; hy, hysteria; pd, psychopathic deviate; pa, paranoia; pt, psychasthenia; sc, schizophrenia; ma, mania. (*From* Vgontzas AN, Lin HM, Papaliaga M, et al. Short sleep duration and obesity: the role of emotional stress and sleep disturbance. Int J Obes 2008;32(5):801–9; with permission.)

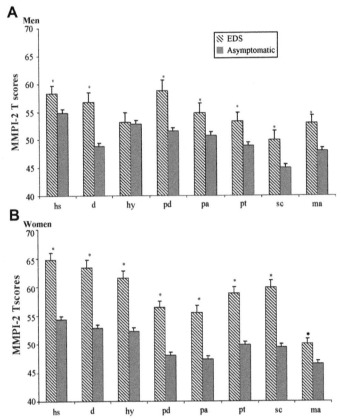

Fig. 4. MMPI profiles in asymptomatic (without sleep disturbance) obese versus obese with EDS (top panel [*A*] men, bottom panel [*B*] women). Mean MMPI-2T scores + 1 standard error in all eight clinical scales after adjustment for age. *P<.05 obese with EDS versus obese with no sleep disturbance. hs, hypochondriasis; d, depression; hy, hysteria; pd, psychopathic deviate; pa, paranoia; pt, psychasthenia; sc, schizophrenia; ma, mania.

effect of sleep complaints on the reduction of self-reported sleep duration was greater in the more distressed subjects than in the less distressed subjects.

DISCUSSION OF KEY FINDINGS

The major finding of our study is that, in a large general population sample, the complaint of

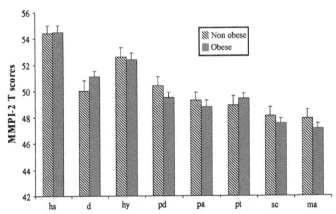

Fig. 5. MMPI profiles in obese versus nonobese without sleep disturbances after adjustment for age and gender. No significant differences were observed. hs, hypochondriasis; d, depression; hy, hysteria; pd, psychopathic deviate; pa, paranoia; pt, psychasthenia; sc, schizophrenia; ma, mania.

a sleep disturbance and chronic emotional stress are the primary predictors of short sleep duration reported by obese subjects.

Many studies have shown that obesity is associated with self-reported short sleep duration[5–11] and it has been assumed that voluntary sleep curtailment is one of the possible mechanisms that lead to obesity. Our study suggests that in the obese, self-reported short sleep duration is not an indication of voluntary sleep restriction but rather is a marker of the presence of subjective sleep disturbances and emotional stress. In contrast, obese subjects without sleep disturbances or emotional stress did not differ in self-reported sleep duration from nonobese controls, suggesting that obesity per se does not contribute significantly to the shorter sleep duration associated with obesity.

In the 1300 subjects from central Pennsylvania, the association between reported sleep duration and BMI was curvilinear with reduced sleep duration associated with increasing BMI consistent with previous studies.[5–8,10,11] Also, a smaller number of subjects slept more than 8 hours. Based on our study, the group of "long sleepers" consists of two subgroups. The first, which is the larger group, consists of nondistressed, older subjects (age >45), an age associated with conditions of prolonged sleep duration and objective EDS, such as sleep apnea and metabolic syndrome,[21–23] and a second group of young, emotionally distressed, obese subjects consistent with previous studies that showed that in the young, depression is frequently associated with hypersomnia or extended periods in bed.[18,24]

Another important finding of our study is that a significantly larger percentage of obese subjects reported sleep complaints compared with nonobese controls (47% vs. 25%). It is possible that obesity and sleep pathology share some common pathophysiologic abnormalities that lead to this significant overlap. Many of the neural systems in the hypothalamus important in sleep/wake regulation, such as CRH, IL6, and orexin, may also play a role in weight maintenance.[25–27] Interestingly, a recent study showed that obesity and sleep pathology, ie, insomnia and sleepiness, share common genetic factors.[28] Also, the increased comorbidity of obesity with medical and psychiatric disorders[29] may lead to the increased prevalence of sleep complaints. However, in our study, depression and pain/discomfort-related disorders were not more prevalent in obese versus nonobese. Independent of the underlying mechanisms, our data suggest that obese subjects are vulnerable to sleep pathology, and evaluation and treatment for their sleep complaints should be part of their multidimensional treatment plan.

Emotional stress was strongly associated with sleep complaints consistent with previous findings in regard to insomnia and EDS.[17,18,30] Interestingly, in a recent study in elderly women, stress related to poor social relations and poor sleep quality had additive effects on plasma interleukin-6 levels, a known marker of increased morbidity and mortality.[31] This suggests that in distressed obese with sleep disturbances, improving both conditions may have additive beneficial effects on their physical as well as emotional health, and longevity.

Our cross-sectional study does not allow for a cause–effect association between stress and obesity. However, it has been suggested that chronic stress leads to the increased consumption of palatable food ("comfort food") and subsequent weight gain and that, in turn, comfort food reduces the activity of the stress system and its attendant anxiety.[32,33] Support for the possibility that consumption of "comfort food" might be a significant factor to the current obesity trend is that between 1971–2000 there has been a significant increase of daily average caloric intake[34] while physical activity levels showed little change.[35] This increase might be related to increased job and social stressors[36] and the drop, in the same period, of the prevalence of common practices that are associated with reduction of perceived stress, eating, and weight, ie, smoking.[37] Smoking reduces eating and weight, and is more prevalent in nonobese subjects, consistent with the data from our. Independent of the direction of the association between stress and obesity, stress management and more healthy coping mechanisms to deal with stress may be very useful in the prevention and treatment of this 47% of the general obese population. In contrast, the same methods may be of no use for the non-distressed 53% of the general obese population.

OBJECTIVE SLEEP DURATION, OBESITY, STRESS, AND SLEEP COMPLAINTS—EPIDEMIOLOGIC SAMPLES

In the same Penn State cohort, we examined the association between objective sleep duration and obesity. Overall, the association of BMI, stress, and sleep complaints with objective sleep duration was weaker compared with self-reported sleep. In a regression analysis where percent sleep time was the outcome variable, MMPI-2 average score and, to a lesser degree, BMI predicted amount of sleep after controlling for age, smoking, and SDB. Specifically, one standard deviation increase of MMPI-2 (7.7 units) was associated with a decrease of 0.7% of percent sleep time ($P<.05$). Also, one standard deviation increase of BMI (6.7 kg/m^2) was associated with a decrease of 0.6% (approximately 3 minutes) of percent sleep time ($P<.1$). In a similar regression analysis that included BMI and sleep complaints as predictors, objective sleep duration was significantly associated with sleep complaints in men. Specifically, in men, the presence of a sleep complaint was associated with a decrease of 3.2% (approximately 15 minutes) of percent sleep time ($P<.05$), whereas for one standard deviation increase of BMI (4.3 kg/m^2), there was a decrease of percent sleep time by 0.5% (NS). In a model that included all three variables, ie, BMI, MMPI-2, and sleep complaints, only sleep complaints were significantly associated with a reduction of percent sleep time ($P<.05$). Finally, SDB was associated with a significant reduction of percent sleep time ($P<.05$).

The lack of a significant association between obesity and objective measures of sleep duration in our study is consistent with two previous studies that reported no association between obesity and objective sleep duration.[7,38] Two more recent studies reported that short sleep duration measured with actigraphy is associated with obesity in elderly community samples. However, in one study, sleep apnea was not assessed objectively and, after controlling for sleep fragmentation, the association was lost,[39] whereas in the second one, after controlling for sleep apnea and total sleep time over the 24-hour period, the association became small and of no clinical or public health significance.[40] That there is no robust association between objective sleep duration and weight suggests that an individual's perception of sleep duration is influenced by factors other than sleep per se, such as sleep complaints as well as emotional stress and social factors.[17,18,41]

OBJECTIVE SLEEP DURATION, OBESITY, AND STRESS—CLINICAL SAMPLES OF MORBIDLY OBESE

In 1994, we reported that morbidly obese men and women, who were tested in the sleep laboratory as part of their comprehensive evaluation before entering a treatment for their obesity and did not show sleep disordered breathing, demonstrated a significant degree of sleep disturbance compared with nonobese controls.[42] Specifically, nighttime sleep duration was shorter, and their sleep was fragmented, ie, increased number of wake time after sleep onset, number of awakenings, and percentage of stage 1 sleep while rapid eye movement sleep was significantly lower.

In 1998, in a subgroup of 73 obese subjects and 45 controls for whom we obtained objective daytime sleep data, we reported that (a) obese sleep more during the day than nonobese, and (b) obese who slept more at night slept also more during the day and vice versa[43] The latter was an unexpected finding which, however, indicated that nighttime sleep disturbance is not the cause of excessive sleep during the day. Similar findings were reported in obese clinical and community samples.[44,45]

To understand further what distinguishes the "long sleepers" from the "short sleepers," in our 73 obese subjects in whom we had both nighttime and daytime polysomnographic measures, we

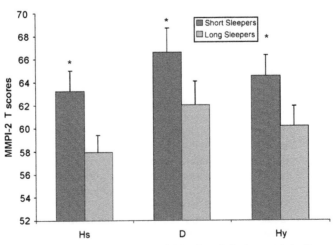

Fig. 6. Obese subjects with short versus long sleep time (objective nighttime and daytime measures) have higher level of psychologic distress. Mean MMPI-2T scores + 1 standard error. *$P<.05$. hs, hypochondriasis; d, depression; hy, hysteria. (*From* Vgontzas AN, Bixler EO, Chrousos GP, et al. Obesity and sleep disturbance: meaningful subtyping of obesity. Arch Physiol Biochem 2008;114(4):224–36; with permission.)

examined whether psychologic distress might play a role in their differential sleep patterns.[46] We divided the obese group into long versus short sleepers based on total sleep time calculated from both the nighttime and daytime sleep data. As a cut-off point, we used the median total sleep time (nighttime and daytime percent sleep). The obese subjects who exhibited shorter sleep had significantly higher scores on three scales of the MMPI (Hypochondriasis [Hs], Depression [D], Hysteria [Hy]) compared with those who demonstrated longer sleep (**Fig. 6**). Thus, it appears that in clinical samples objective short sleep time in a 24-hour sleep–wake cycle is associated with higher levels of psychologic distress. It is also possible that in this morbidly obese clinical population, sleep complaints are more frequent and more severe compared with obese individuals in the general population. The role of stress and sleep complaints in predicting objective short sleep in morbidly obese is supported further by that in two experimental studies by our group, severely obese volunteer subjects who were carefully selected not to have poor sleep or to be distressed, slept at night as well as nonobese subjects.[27,47]

More recently, studies have shown that in the presence of a sleep complaint, ie, insomnia or "poor sleep," objective sleep duration is a predictor of cardiometabolic morbidity.[48] Thus, objective short sleep duration in the morbidly obese with sleep complaints may predict higher cardiometabolic risks, ie, worsened obesity, hypertension, diabetes, and improving both the quality and quantity of sleep in these individuals may be important.

CONCLUSIONS

Our data suggest that in obese individuals, subjective short sleep duration is associated with frequent sleep complaints and increased levels of stress. This view is supported by more recent data that suggest an association of subjective sleep duration with social stress and unhealthy daytime behaviors.

For example, longitudinal data from the Alameda County Health and Living Study indicated that short sleep duration is also influenced by social stressors such as socioeconomic and minority status.[49] Furthermore, in a report by the Centers for Disease Control and Prevention released in May 2008, Schoenborn and Adams[50] provide a national perspective on the association between sleep duration and selected health risk behaviors using data from the 2004–2006 National Health Interview Survey. The findings suggested that United States adults who usually sleep less than 6 hours were more likely than adults who slept 7 to 8 hours to engage in certain health risk behaviors (ie, cigarette smoking, consuming five or more alcoholic drinks per day, and not engaging in physical activity during leisure time). Finally, Stamatakis and Brownson[51] reported that short sleep duration is associated with less physical activity and lower fruit and vegetable consumption.

This emerging literature suggests that obese individuals who report short sleep are psychosocially stressed and unhappy with the quality of their sleep, and engage in unhealthy behaviors, such as increased consumption of palatable (or "comfort") food[29] or reduced physical activity, which may lead to excess weight. Furthermore, behaviors such as smoking and alcohol consumption are widely used to reduce stress and to improve, albeit unsuccessfully, sleep, whereas their discontinuation, eg, smoking, is associated with increased food intake and significant weight gain. Thus, from a practical standpoint it appears that the self-reported short sleep duration is a marker of subjective sleep disturbances and their associated chronic psychosocial stress and unhealthy wake-time behaviors.

In addition, objective short sleep duration in the presence of a sleep complaint or stress is strongly associated with cardiometabolic risk factors, ie, hypertension and diabetes, compared with either problem alone. Thus, objective short sleep duration may be a very useful measure in predicting clinical severity and morbidity, such as hypertension, diabetes, and obesity.

Sleeping better, reducing or coping with chronic stress more effectively, and promoting healthier behaviors appear to be very important for a significant percentage (almost 50%) of obese individuals in the general population of the United States. In some instances, ie, obese with sleep complaints and short objective sleep duration, lengthening their objective sleep may be an important aspect of their treatment. However, simply recommending to poor sleepers to lengthen their sleep by 1 or 2 hours may be countertherapeutic.

SUMMARY

Short sleep duration and sleep loss have been suggested as novel risk factors that may lead to obesity, a condition where prevalence has reached such levels to be considered epidemic and a major public health problem. One important question that has received little attention is what people mean when they respond to "how many hours do you sleep on the average." It appears that the number of self-reported hours of sleep is more strongly associated with the quality of sleep and less with its measured quantity. In the Penn State cohort of 1741 men and women, we showed that self-reported short sleep duration is associated with more sleep complaints and emotional stress, and less with objective sleep duration. These data are consistent with other studies that report weak or no association between measured sleep and obesity. Furthermore, other studies show that self-reported short sleep duration in obese is associated with low socioeconomic and minority status, cigarette smoking, alcohol use, low physical activity, and unhealthy diet.

Does this mean that measured sleep is of no use in our fight against obesity? Morbidly obese patients, particularly those who are distressed, appear to sleep objectively less compared with healthy nonobese. Furthermore, among patients with poor sleep, those with short objective sleep have worse outcomes in terms of severity and cardiometabolic morbidity. Thus, objective measures of sleep may be very useful in detecting these individuals at high risk for medical morbidity frequently associated with obesity, ie, hypertension, diabetes, and so forth.

From a practical standpoint, self-reported sleep duration may serve to detect subjective sleep complaints, psychosocial stress, and unhealthy behaviors, which should be the focus of our preventive and therapeutic strategies for obesity. Further studies are needed to confirm the promising role of objective measures of sleep in predicting cardiometabolic morbidity among patients with sleep complaints.

REFERENCES

1. Flegal KM, Carroll MD, Ogden CL, et al. Prevalence and trends in obesity among US adults, 1999–2000. JAMA 2002;288(14):1723–7.
2. Spiegel A, Nabel E, Volkow N, et al. Obesity on the brain. Nat Neurosci 2005;8(5):552–3.
3. Tune GS. Sleep and wakefulness in normal human adults. Br Med J 1968;2(5600):269–71.
4. National Sleep Foundation. 2005 Sleep in America Poll. Washington, DC: National Sleep Foundation; 2005.
5. Kripke DF, Garfinkel L, Wingard DL, et al. Mortality associated with sleep duration and insomnia. Arch Gen Psychiatry 2002;59(2):131–6.
6. Gottlieb DJ, Redline S, Nieto FJ, et al. Association of usual sleep duration with hypertension: the Sleep Heart Health Study. Sleep 2006;29(8):1009–14.
7. Taheri S, Lin L, Austin D, et al. Short sleep duration is associated with reduced leptin, elevated ghrelin, and increased body mass index. PLoS Med 2004; 1(3):210–7.
8. Kohatsu ND, Tsai R, Young T, et al. Sleep duration and body mass index in a rural population. Arch Intern Med 2006;166(16):1701–5.
9. Vorona RD, Winn MP, Babineau TW, et al. Overweight and obese patients in a primary care population report less sleep than patients with a normal body mass index. Arch Intern Med 2005;165(1):25–30.
10. Gangwisch JE, Malaspina D, Boden-Albala B, et al. Inadequate sleep as a risk factor for obesity: analyses of the NHANES I. Sleep 2005;28(10):1289–96.
11. Hasler G, Buysse DJ, Klaghofer R, et al. The association between short sleep duration and obesity in young adults: a 13-year prospective study. Sleep 2004;27(4):661–6.
12. Spiegel K, Leproult R, van Cauter E. Impact of sleep debt on metabolic land endocrine function. Lancet 1999;354(9188):1435–9.
13. Spiegel K, Leproult R, Colecchia EF, et al. Adaptation of the 24-h growth hormone profile to a state of sleep debt. Am J Physiol Regul Integr Comp Physiol 2000;279(3):R874–83.
14. Lauderdale DS, Knutson KL, Yan LL, et al. Self-reported and measured sleep duration. How similar are they? Epidemiology 2008;19(6):838–45.
15. Vgontzas AN, Lin HM, Papaliaga M, et al. Short sleep duration and obesity: the role of emotional stress and sleep disturbance. Int J Obes 2008; 32(5):801–9.
16. Butcher JN, Dahlstrom WG, Graham JR, et al. Manual for the standardized Minnesota Multiphasic Personality Inventory: MMPI-2. An administrative and interpretive guide. Minneapolis (MN): University of Minnesota Press; 1989.
17. Bixler EO, Vgontzas AN, Lin HM, et al. Insomnia in central Pennsylvania. J Psychosom Res 2002; 53(1):589–92.
18. Bixler EO, Vgontzas AN, Lin HM, et al. Excessive daytime sleepiness in a general population sample: the role of sleep apnea, age, obesity, diabetes and depression. J Clin Endocrinol Metab 2005;9(8): 4510–5.
19. Kuczmarski RJ, Flegal KM, Campbell SM, et al. Increasing prevalence of overweight among US adults. The National Health and Nutrition Examination Surveys, 1960 to 1991. JAMA 1994;272(3): 205–11.
20. Kuczmarski RJ, Flegal KM. Criteria for definition of overweight in transition: background and recommendations for the United States. Am J Clin Nutr 2000;72(5):1074–81.
21. Bixler EO, Vgontzas AN, Ten Have T, et al. Effects of age on sleep apnea in men: I. Prevalence and severity. Am J Respir Crit Care Med 1998;157(1): 144–8.
22. Bixler EO, Vgontzas AN, Lin HM, et al. Prevalence of sleep-disordered breathing in women. Am J Respir Crit Care Med 2001;163(3):608–13.

23. Young T, Palta M, Dempsey J, et al. The occurrence of sleep-disordered breathing among middle-aged adults. N Engl J Med 1993;328(17):1230–5.

24. American Psychiatric Association. Diagnostic and statistical manual of mental disorders. Washington, DC: American Psychiatric Association; 1994.

25. Flier SJ, Elmquist JK. A good night's sleep: future antidote to the obesity epidemic? Ann Intern Med 2004;141(11):885–6.

26. Chrousos GP. The role of stress and the hypothalamic-pituitary-adrenal axis in the pathogenesis of the metabolic syndrome: neuron-endocrine and target tissue-related causes. Int J Obes Relat Metab Disord 2000;24(Suppl 2):S50–5.

27. Vgontzas AN, Papanicolaou DA, Bixler EO, et al. Sleep apnea and daytime sleepiness and fatigue: relation to visceral obesity, insulin resistance, and hypercytokinemia. J Clin Endocrinol Metab 2000; 85(3):1151–8.

28. Watson NF, Goldberg J, Arguelles L, et al. Genetic and environmental influences on insomnia, daytime sleepiness, and obesity in twins. Sleep 2006;29(5):645–9.

29. Stunkard AJ, Faith MS, Allison KC. Depression and obesity. Biol Psychiatry 2003;54(3):330–7.

30. Buysse DJ, Reynolds CF III, Kupfer DJ, et al. Clinical diagnoses in 216 insomnia patients using the ICSD and proposed DSM-IV and ICD-10 categories: a report from the APA/NIMH DSM-IV field trials. Sleep 1994;17(7):630–7.

31. Friedman EM, Hayney MS, Love GD, et al. Social relationships, sleep quality, and interleukin-6 in aging women. Proc Natl Acad Sci U S A 2005; 102(51):18757–62.

32. Dallman MF, Pecoraro N, Akana SF, et al. Chronic stress and obesity: a new view of "comfort food". Proc Natl Acad Sci U S A 2003;100(20):11696–701.

33. Pecoraro N, Reyes F, Gomez F, et al. Chronic stress promotes palatable feeding, which reduces signs of stress: feedforward and feedback effects of chronic stress. Endocrinology 2004;145(8):3754–62.

34. Centers for Disease Control and Prevention. Trends in intake of energy and macronutrients – United States, 1971–2000. MMWR Morb Mortal Wkly Rep 2004;53(4):80–2.

35. Centers for Disease Control and Prevention. Physical activity trends – United States, 1990–1998. MMWR Morb Mortal Wkly Rep 2001;50(9):166–9.

36. Nishitani N, Sakakibara H. Relationship of obesity to job stress and eating behavior in male Japanese workers. Int J Obes 2006;30(3):528–33.

37. Williamson DF. Weight change in middle-aged Americans. Am J Prev Med 2004;27(1):81–2.

38. Lauderdale DS, Knutson KL, Yan LL, et al. Objectively measured sleep characteristics among early-middle-

aged adults: the CARDIA study. Am J Epidemiol 2006;164:5–16.

39. van den Berg JF, Knvistingh Neven A, Tulen JH, et al. Actigraphic sleep duration and fragmentation are related to obesity in the elderly: the Rotterdam Study. Int J Obes 2008;32(7):1083–90.

40. Patel SR, Blackwell T, Redline S, et al. The association between sleep duration and obesity in older adults. Int J Obes 2008;32(12):1825–34.

41. Bliwise DL, Young TB. The parable of parabola: what the U-shaped curve can and cannot tell us about sleep. Sleep 2007;30(12):1614–5.

42. Vgontzas AN, Tan TL, Bixler EO, et al. Sleep apnea and sleep disruption in obese patients. Arch Intern Med 1994;154(15):1705–11.

43. Vgontzas AN, Bixler EO, Tan TL, et al. Obesity without sleep apnea is associated with daytime sleepiness. Arch Intern Med 1998;158(12):1333–7.

44. Resta O, Foschino-Barbaro MP, Legari G, et al. Sleep-related breathing disorders, loud snoring and excessive daytime sleepiness in obese subjects. Int J Obes Relat Metab Disord 2001;25(5):669–75.

45. Punjabi NM, O'hearn DJ, Neubauer DN, et al. Modeling hypersomnolence in sleep-disordered breathing. A novel approach using survival analysis. Am J Respir Crit Care Med 1999;159(6):1703–9.

46. Vgontzas AN, Bixler EO, Chrousos GP, et al. Obesity and sleep disturbance: meaningful sub-typing of obesity. Arch Physiol Biochem 2008;114(4):224–36.

47. Vgontzas AN, Pejovic S, Zoumakis E, et al. Hypothalamic–pituitary–adrenal axis activity in obese men with and without sleep apnea: effects of continuous positive airway pressure therapy. J Clin Endocrinol Metab 2007;92(11):4199–207.

48. Vgontzas AN, Liao D, Bixler EO, et al. Insomnia with objective short sleep duration is associated with a high risk for hypertension. Sleep (in press).

49. Stamatakis KA, Kaplan GA, Roberts RE. Short sleep duration across income, education and race/ethnic groups: population prevalence and growing disparities during 34 years of follow-up. Ann Epidemiol 2007;17(12):948–55.

50. Schoenborn CA, Adams PF. Sleep duration as a correlate of smoking, alcohol use, leisure-time physical inactivity, and obesity among adults: United States, 2004–2006. Department of Health and Human Services, Center for Disease control and Prevention. National Center for Health Statistics. Available at: http://www.cdc/gov/nchs/products/pubs/pubd/hestats/sleep04-06/sleep04-06.htm. Accessed May, 2008.

51. Stamatakis KA, Brownson RC. Sleep duration and obesity-related risk factors in the rural Midwest. Prev Med 2008;46(5):439–44.

Sleep Patterns in the Transition from Adolescence to Young Adulthood

Antonio Vela-Bueno, MD*, Julio Fernandez-Mendoza, PsyD,
Sara Olavarrieta-Bernardino, PsyD

KEYWORDS

- Young adults • Sleep habits • Sleepiness
- Sleep disorders • Academic performance

The transition between adolescence and adulthood takes place between 18 and 25 years, with different authors identifying varying ranges of age.[1] Factors that may contribute to prolonging (eg, graduate education) or to shortening (eg, early marriage) this duration may contribute to that variability.

Generally speaking, despite the relevant maturational and developmental changes that take place during this transitional period, this period of life has received relatively little attention compared with childhood or adolescence.[2]

Sleep and sleep-related health issues in this period of life also have received relatively little attention, despite the presence of sleep complaints and disorders.[3] A recent review article on the health status of young adults (age 18–24 years) in the United States completely ignored sleep.[4] It included alcohol as a causative factor in driving accidents, but it did not mention sleep, although sleep-related crashes are common in this population. For example, in a study in North Carolina,[5] 55% of motor vehicle accidents that resulted from the driver's falling asleep at the wheel (a common manifestation of daytime sleepiness) involved people 25 years of age or younger, with the peak age of occurrence being 20 years of age.

Developmental changes, rather than maturational ones, seem to have an important role in some of the main sleep complaints in this period of life. These complaints include disturbances of the sleep–wakefulness circadian rhythm, insufficient sleep, and the resulting excessive daytime sleepiness.

This article first reviews the developmental and maturational changes associated with normal and disturbed sleep and continues with a review of the epidemiologic data on sleep complaints and disorders during the transition from adolescence to adulthood. The existing data come mainly from college student populations. The last section makes some recommendations for prevention of and coping with sleep disturbances.

MATURATIONAL AND DEVELOPMENTAL CHANGES

In the late years of adolescence and in the early years of adulthood some maturational processes are still being completed, whereas a slow decline of some functions starts to occur in young adults even in their early 20s.[2] Generally speaking, there is some overlap between progression and regression in the transition from adolescence to adulthood.

The sleep pattern of young adults has been used as a template to assess the changes in sleep along the life cycle.[6] Nevertheless a more nuanced description of sleep patterns in more specific age subgroups of young adulthood, including the transition between adolescence and adulthood, is lacking.

Human Sleep and Applied Chronobiology Laboratory, Department of Psychiatry, Universidad Autonoma de Madrid, c/Arzobispo Morcillo, 4, 28029 Madrid, Spain
* Corresponding author.
E-mail address: antonio.vela@uam.es (A. Vela-Bueno).

Sleep Med Clin 4 (2009) 77–85
doi:10.1016/j.jsmc.2008.12.003

To ascertain the sleep changes in this period, comparisons with bordering age groups must be used. This section describes the differences between the age groups of 16 to 19 years (mean age: females, 17.3 years; males, 17.4 years), 13 to 15 years (mean age: females, 14.1 years; males, 14.0 years), and 20 to 29 years (mean age: females, 24.5 years; males, 24.3 years). The data are from a study assessing sleep measures in subjects ranging in age from 3 to 79 years.[7] The main differences between groups are summarized in **Boxes 1** and **2**.

Some general changes in the sleep patterns in individuals during the transition from adolescence to adulthood are a decrease in the total time spent in bed, in the total sleep period, and in total sleep time. These decreases are observed in older adolescents (age, 16 to 19 years) as compared with younger adolescents (age, 13 to 15 years). For slow-wave sleep and REM sleep the evolution is not homogeneous. The percentage of REM sleep decreases in older adolescents of both sexes as compared with younger adolescents, but no differences are found in slow-wave sleep. When compared with older adolescent females, young adult women (age, 20 to 29 years) show a decrease in the percentage of slow-wave sleep, whereas young adult men have a decrease in rapid-eye-movement (REM) sleep as compared with older adolescent males.[7]

In general, during the transition from adolescence to adulthood changes in sleep occur that indicate the end of maturation and the beginning of adulthood. Most of these changes, in an

---

Box 1
Significant differences in sleep architecture in older (age, 16 to 19 years) and younger (age, 13 to 15 years) adolescents

Females

Older adolescent females spent a smaller percentage of the sleep time period in rapid-eye-movement (REM) sleep and had a longer interval between the third and fourth REM sleep periods than younger adolescent females

Males

Older adolescent males spent less time in bed, had shorter sleep periods and total sleep time, had fewer REM periods, and spent a smaller percentage of the sleep time period in REM sleep than younger adolescent males.

Data from Williams RL, Karacan I, Hursch CJ. EEG of human sleep: clinical applications. New York: John Wiley & Sons; 1974. p. 48.

Box 2
Significant differences in sleep architecture in young adults (age, 20 to 29 years) and older adolescents (age, 16 to 19 years)

Females

Adult women spent less time in bed, had shorter sleep periods and total sleep times, had shorter REM latency, and spent a lower percentage of the sleep time period in stage 4 and slow-wave sleep than older adolescent females

Males

Adult males spent less time in bed, had shorter sleep periods and total sleep times, had shorter REM latency, and spent a greater percentage of the sleep period time in REM sleep than older adolescent males.

Data from Williams RL, Karacan I, Hursch CJ. EEG of human sleep: clinical applications. New York: John Wiley & Sons; 1974. p. 49.

---

attenuated way, are similar to the more marked changes observed with more advanced aging.

From a developmental standpoint, changes occur in this period of life that can have both direct and indirect effects on sleep habits. Those changes are related mainly to the individuation process and to the occupational and social challenges typical of this age.

From an individuation standpoint, this is the time of separation (both intrapsychic and real) from parents, when parental guidance gives way to autonomy, with the young person making decisions about his/her life patterns, including sleep habits that frequently are incompatible with adequate sleep hygiene. In terms of the individuation process this period is when societal influences have the most important role in shaping the individual's personality.[1] In some instances these societal influences may represent a source of pressure (eg, peer pressure).

This period is the time of starting college and/or work. In college students, the stress from academic demands may have a negative impact on sleep,[8] and the need to adjust the sleep schedule to the school schedule may contribute to restricted sleep time. Another source of stress can be the need to manage work and family life in the minority of individuals who create a family during this age period.

In summary, the transition from adolescence to adulthood involves several new sources of stress and the need to adjust the sleep–wakefulness schedules to the new occupational and social conditions. These challenges can have negative consequences on sleep and increase the likelihood of sleep complaints.

SLEEP COMPLAINTS AND DISORDERS

Individuals in the transition from adolescence to adulthood may present with any type of sleep complaint or disorder, including those that are more typical of previous and subsequent stages of the life cycle. Some complaints, however, seem to be found more frequently among adolescents and young adults. Several recent epidemiologic studies have shown that excessive daytime sleepiness is quite common among young adults.[9–11] In a study from the authors' group,[12] based on a population of first-year university students, 29.6% had a score above 10 on the Epworth Sleepiness Scale (ESS), which suggests the existence of meaningful sleepiness.[13] Similar figures with the ESS have been found by other authors.[14]

Some primary disorders of excessive sleepiness (eg, narcolepsy, idiopathic hypersomnia, and some periodic hypersomnias) have a peak in the age of onset in the second and the third decades,[15] but their limited prevalence cannot explain the findings in the epidemiologic studies cited previously. It is generally accepted[16] that the main cause of excessive daytime sleepiness is insufficient sleep, which is a common finding both in clinical practice and in epidemiologic studies.[16] Chronic sleep restriction seems to be common among individuals in this age group[9] and results from poor sleep hygiene, which in these individuals is an outcome of the developmental changes mentioned earlier.

The main direct causative factors of insufficient sleep in general are too little time allowed for sleep, irregularities in the sleep–wakefulness schedule, and delays of the sleep phase. The next sections focus on sleep habits, circadian disturbances, and insufficient sleep. They also discuss napping, a common behavior in this age cohort.

SLEEP HABITS

It is a widespread health concern that adolescents and young adults frequently adopt habits that are not compatible with good sleep. Among the inadequate sleep hygiene practices are irregularity of schedule and inadequate napping, habitual use of sleep-disturbing substances such as alcohol, caffeine, or nicotine, and engaging in physically activating, emotionally upsetting, or mentally stimulating activities, especially in the period preceding bedtime.[15] There are few detailed descriptions in the literature of these activities in

the young. The authors assessed the sleep-related habits and behaviors in a population of first-year university students attending one of the main universities in Madrid, Spain. There were 1271 sample subjects including both sexes, with a mean age of 18.9 years (range, 16–25 years). The detailed methodology of this study has been published elsewhere.[12] One section of the survey included questions about the activities in which the subjects engaged during the pre-bedtime period. These activities did not need to be mutually exclusive, and the subjects could do more than one activity in that period of time. The most frequently reported activities were (by order of frequency) watching television, reading, and listening music. All these activities could be considered neutral, with their affective valence and their arousing potential depending on the content and the context. In contrast, other frequently reported activities can have a well-defined arousing effect, such as using the computer (42.4% of the subjects), studying (36.7%), or doing the homework (27%). Other sleep-disturbing behaviors, such as drinking alcohol or caffeine or smoking, also are included in **Table 1**.

The bedtimes of the subjects showed a marked difference between weekdays and weekends (**Fig. 1**). Although more than 96% of the students went to bed before 2 AM on weekdays, fewer than 20% did so during the weekends, with about two thirds of the participants going to bed between 2 AM and 5 AM and a substantial percentage (19.4%) going to bed later than 5 AM. Nearly 80% of the subjects got up before 9 AM on weekdays, whereas more than 75% awakened between 10 AM and 2 AM on weekends, and 7.5%

Table 1 Self-reported activities in the pre-bedtime period	
Activity	**%**
Watching television	85.6
Reading	53.0
Listening to music	52.3
Using the computer	42.4
Studying	36.8
Eating	23.2
Drinking dairy products	22.4
Drinking soft drinks	22.4
Doing homework	20.0
Smoking	8.2
Drinking alcohol	4.0

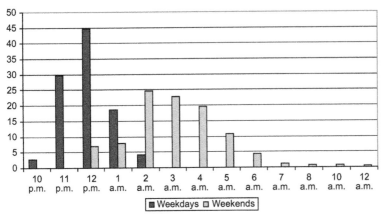

Fig. 1. Self-reported bedtimes on both weekdays and weekends. Bars represent the percentage of students reporting the various bedtimes.

* Bars represent the percentage of students reporting the various bedtimes

awakened between 2 and 6 PM. This figure, added to the 25.6% that arose between noon and 2 PM, point to a high prevalence of extended sleep over the weekend. In general, this pattern suggests that a remarkable number of students undergo a circadian desynchronization during the weekend. Because of its resemblance to jet lag, this sleep pattern has been named "social jet lag."[17] Similar findings have been reported repeatedly in various publications.[18–20]

The self-reported sleep latency of the subjects during the week was moderately longer than normal values (27 minutes) and was shorter on weekends (15 minutes), probably reflecting a certain recovery from weekday sleep restriction. Despite the quasi-normality of these sleep latency values, a substantial proportion of the participants (28%) complained of difficulty initiating sleep; this difficulty can be related to the delay of the sleep phase, as discussed in the next section.

CIRCADIAN RHYTHM DISORDERS

Circadian rhythm disorders have in common a mismatch between the individual's sleep–wakefulness rhythm and the physical and social environment.[15] Therefore sleep occurs at times that are undesirable for the subject. For this article, the subtypes most relevant are the delayed sleep phase type or syndrome (DSPS) and the irregular sleep–wake type (ISWT).

The DSPS is characterized by a markedly delayed sleep onset (which is stable with little day-to-day variation), typically occurring between 2 and 6 AM, and a wake time that takes place in the late morning or afternoon.[15] Sleep duration, architecture, and quality are normal if the individuals are allowed to follow their preferred schedule. If, however, they try to fall asleep and wake up at times that are compatible with societal demands

(eg, work or school), the results are a marked difficulty initiating sleep at night, excessive sleepiness and even "sleep drunkenness" (extreme difficulty awakening and confusion) in the morning, and excessive sleepiness and the associated deficits during the day. In other words, the individuals suffer sustained partial sleep deprivation on weekdays; in contrast, on weekends and holidays, they try to compensate by oversleeping while going to bed at their preferred times (ie, a marked expression of "social jet lag").[17] DSPS is considered to be most prevalent among adolescents and young adults, with a mean age of onset of 20 years.[15] In general the reported prevalence for those ages range between 7% and 16%,[15] with one study reporting a prevalence of 17% in college students.[21]

A distinction needs to be made between DSPS per se and "motivated sleep phase delay,"[22] which is related to social, psychologic, and behavioral factors and can be considered volitional in nature. Without such a distinction the figures for DSPS are overinflated. In general there is trend to over-report sleep delays. Thus 30.2% of the authors' subjects reported DSPS, although 96% of them went to bed earlier than 2 AM on weekdays. One study that used strict criteria and made such a distinction found much lower rates of prevalence in a Norwegian population.[23] The ages of these subjects ranged from 18 to 67 years. The prevalence in the total sample was 0.17%, whereas in the group aged 18 and 19 years the prevalence was 0.34%, and the prevalence of motivated sleep phase delay was 4.6%.

The consequences of the sleep-phase delays, motivated or not, are mainly those of the chronic partial sleep deprivation, with the addition of the consequences of temporal mismatch. They have negative effects on occupational performance, interpersonal relationships, and social commitments.

In its most severe forms ISWT is characterized by the lack of a clearly defined circadian rhythm of sleep and wakefulness.[15] There is a disorganization of the sleep and wakefulness periods so that they vary throughout the 24 hours, and the individuals may complain of insomnia and/or excessive sleepiness, with naps being taken commonly. One of the main predisposing factors is poor sleep hygiene,[15] and milder forms can be found in subjects who have inadequate habits, as do many young individuals. The prevalence is not well understood. In the authors' sample, 8.4% of the subjects reported having an irregular pattern. It has been shown that having an irregular pattern is associated with daytime sleepiness in students who are not sleep deprived.[24] Also, a recent study showed a decrement in performance in medical students who have an irregular sleep–wake cycle.[25]

In summary, irregularities and delays of the sleep phase are common among young individuals. These irregularities cause and increase the effects of insufficient sleep.

INSUFFICIENT SLEEP

Insufficient sleep seems to be a common finding among individuals in the transition between adolescence and young adulthood, as shown by several recent studies.[26–29] One study[26] obtained self-reported data from questionnaires administered to 1412 students at a Korean university. The mean sleep duration of the respondents was 6.7 hours, with 30.2% reporting insufficient sleep; about one third of them mentioned the use of visual media (including computers) as the main reason for the lack of sleep, but no distinction was made between school and nonschool days.

Ninety-three percent of the students were between the ages of 19 and 24 years. Two studies done in Taiwan, although reporting short sleep in students, found differences between school days and nonschool days or between weekdays versus weekends. In the first study,[27] in a sample of 1922 first-year college students (average age, 18.5 years), by far the most common sleep complaint was insufficient sleep (23.9%). The average total sleep time was 6 hours and 24 minutes for school days and 8 hours and 27 minutes for nonschool days. In the other study,[28] the subjects were 237 university students (110 women and 127 men) between the ages of 19 and 24 years. In both men and women, significant differences between weekdays and weekends were found in total nighttime sleep and total sleep time in 24 hours, with greater values on weekends.

In a recent worldwide study[29] 17,465 university students aged 17 to 30 years (no mean age was provided) from 24 countries were asked about their sleep time during the 24 hours, with no distinction being made between weekdays and weekends. The lowest mean sleep durations were those of subjects from the four Asian countries represented: Japan (6.20 hours), Korea (6.80), Taiwan (6.61), and Thailand (6.95). This finding suggests some sociocultural influence on the total amount of sleep obtained. Of the total number of subjects in this study who responded, 21% slept less than 7 hours (6% slept less than 6 hours), and short sleep was associated with a poorer self-reported health status.

In the authors' study, the difference in sleep time between weekdays and weekends was about 1 hour (7.5 versus 8.5, respectively). A construct that reflects better the insufficiency of sleep is one the authors have reported as "perceived sleep

Table 2
Sleepiness and fatigue measures associated with increased perceived sleep debt (PSD) among young adults

Measure	N (%)	Associated PSD[a]
Epworth sleepiness scale score >10	368 (29.6)	2:00 ± 1:13[b]
Fatigue	180 (14)	1:30 ± 1:02
Napping	558 (44.4)	1:46 ± 1:14[b]
Missing class because of oversleeping	240 (19)	2:00 ± 1:20[b]
Missing class because of tiredness	315 (25.1)	1:51 ± 1:17[b]
Feeling the need to sleep in class	1037 (82.5)	1:45 ± 1:12[b]
Falling asleep in class	87 (7)	2:03 ± 1:16[b]
Diurnal sleep attacks	195 (15.4)	2:07 ± 1:22[b]
Restlessness in class	560 (46)	1:46 ± 1:11[b]

[a] Values are presented as unadjusted mean ± SD in a hours:minutes format.
[b] Significant at $P < .05$.

Table 3
Napping among young adults

Time of Napping	Prevalence N (%)	Duration[a]
Morning	30 (5.4)	58.79 ± 34.39
Noon	44 (8)	46.32 ± 23.94
Postprandial or early afternoon	501 (90)	72.61 ± 41.78
Late afternoon or evening	66 (12)	90.58 ± 47.91

[a] Values are presented as unadjusted mean ± SD in minutes.

debt" (PSD).[30] The PSD is obtained by calculating the difference between the desired amount of sleep and the actual amount obtained. Both on weekdays and weekends, the subjects' PSD was almost the same (1 hour and 40 minutes and 1 hour and 38 minutes, respectively). The extent to which PSD seems to be associated with various expressions of excessive daytime sleepiness and fatigue is reflected in **Table 2**. One of the behaviors associated with insufficient sleep is napping.

NAPPING

A nap is defined as "any sleep period with a duration of less than 50% of the average major sleep period of an individual."[31] Several types of naps are distinguished according to their purpose:[32] recuperative (taken after an insufficient nighttime sleep), prophylactic (occurring in anticipation of reduced nocturnal sleep), and appetitive (taken for pleasure and/or as part of a semi-circadian rhythm with a maximum in the early afternoon).

Napping is very common among young adult individuals.[25,33–36] In the authors' sample 44% of the subjects reported taking naps;[15] in 90% of the cases naps occurred after lunch, and the mean duration of these naps was longer than 1 hour (**Table 3**). The authors' data and those from other studies point to the recuperative nature of those naps as a way of coping with insufficient sleep.[12,27] Also an association between napping and having an irregular sleep–wakefulness pattern has been documented in the authors' study and in others.[15,36] **Table 4** includes the correlates of napping in the authors' sample.

In summary, young individuals take frequent and long naps of a recuperative nature, most commonly after lunch. Subjects who take naps are more likely to show irregular sleep–wakefulness schedules.

Table 4
Correlates of napping among young adults

Correlate	Odds Ratio (95.0% Confidence Interval)
Irregular sleep pattern	4.37 (2.63–7.26)[c]
Morning college schedule	3.58 (2.60–4.94)[c]
Male gender	1.81 (1.39–2.36)[c]
Diurnal sleep attacks	1.62 (1.13–2.32)[b]
Missing classes because of tiredness	1.60 (1.20–2.15)[c]
Less ability to concentrate during first hour in the afternoon	1.34 (1.04–1.72)[a]
Low depth of nighttime sleep	0.80 (0.66–0.98)[a]
Irritability	0.75 (0.58–0.97)[a]
Less ability to concentrate during second hour in the afternoon	0.69 (0.50–0.96)[a]
Muscular pain	0.55 (0.36–0.83)[b]
Epworth Sleepiness Scale score < 10	0.51 (0.39–0.68)[c]
Difficulty staying asleep	0.49 (0.29–0.82)[b]

[a] $P < .05$.
[b] $P < .01$.
[c] $P < .001$.

Table 5
Duration-dependent effects of naps on daytime functioning and nighttime sleep

Effect	Brief Nap	Long NAP
Alertness and performance	Improvement	Improvement
Duration of improvement	Up to 3 hours	More than 3 hours
Sleep inertia	No	Yes
Disruption of subsequent sleep	No	Yes
Benefits	As effective as a long nap when sleep is normal or restricted	More effective than a short nap after a total sleep deprivation

Data from Brooks A, Lack L. Naps. In: Kushida CA, editor. Sleep deprivation: clinical issues, pharmacology and sleep loss effects. New York: Marcel Dekker; 2005. p. 470–1.

RECOMMENDATIONS

The general recommendations of sleep hygiene also apply for the individuals in this age group. Some of these recommendations need to be emphasized because of the frequency with which this population engages in unhealthy habits.

The most commonly found sleep–wakefulness problems in the period between adolescence and adulthood are those related to the changes in the sleep–wakefulness schedule throughout the week and especially over the weekend. Therefore the first recommendation is to maintain regularity, with some flexibility during the weekends (with bedtimes and wake times being delayed no more than 2 hours) to accommodate the need for socializing that persons have at this age. As a corollary the young people should be encouraged to obtain an optimal amount of sleep both on weekdays and weekends.

Another important issue is that of adequate napping to counteract the effects of insufficient sleep and, at the same time, to avoid irregularity. Table 5 summarizes the effects of naps on subsequent state depending on their duration. There is considerable experimental evidence demonstrating that naps of varying length, including those of a brief duration (< 20 minutes), have positive effects on daytime somnolence and on cognitive functions and performance in healthy subjects (partially sleep deprived or not) in the transition from adolescence to young adulthood.[37–42] Thus in subjects who are slightly or moderately sleep deprived a short nap may be sufficient for a recovery of the functions involved in alertness and performance. Longer naps are needed to compensate for more severe sleep loss. A recent study showed that after a night of sleep loss a 2-hour nap taken between 2 and 4 PM, in addition to decreasing sleepiness and improving performance, caused beneficial changes in cortisol and interleukin-6 secretion in a group of young adults.[43]

From a circadian standpoint, naps taken in the early to mid-afternoon period are the most recuperative.[38] This phenomenon can be explained by the temporal association of the nap with the postlunch dip.

There also are individual differences related to the habit of taking naps. Thus, habitual nappers obtain more benefits from naps than nonnappers.[38,41]

People in this age cohort frequently engage in arousing and/or sleep-disruptive behaviors before bedtime. These activities should be discouraged during this time. **Box 3** includes a summary of the sleep hygiene recommendations for this age group. The two main goals are to maintain regularity and to avoid insufficient sleep.

Through awareness campaigns both health professionals and academic authorities can help increase young persons' understanding of the importance of sleep for good general health and good performance. A few studies have shown that inadequate sleep is associated with poorer

Box 3
Main tips for sleep hygiene in the young

Obtain an adequate amount of sleep

Nap properly

- Take a short nap in the early afternoon
- Avoid multiple naps
- Avoid long naps

Maintain regularity of the sleep–wakefulness schedule

Avoid "social jetlag"

Avoid arousing activities near bedtime (eg, using computers, studying)

Avoid sleep-disrupting substances (eg, alcohol, caffeine) especially near bedtime

Exercise regularly but not close to bedtime

school performance.[44,45] Academic planners also could allow more time for sleep on weekdays by postponing the time that classes start.

REFERENCES

1. Adatto CP. Late adolescence to early adulthood. In: Greenspan SI, Pollock GH, editors. The course of life: psychoanalytic contributions toward understanding personality development. vol II: Latency, adolescence and youth. Bethesda (MD): NIMH; 1980. p. 463–76.

2. Colarusso CA. Adulthood. In: Sadock BJ, Sadock VA, editors. Kaplan and Shadock's comprehensive textbook of psychiatry. 8th edition, vol 2. Philadelphia: Lippincott Williams & Wilkins; 2005. p. 3565–86.

3. Bijwadia J, Dexter D. The student with sleep complaints. In: Lee-Chiong T, editor. Sleep: a comprehensive handbook. Hoboken (NJ): John Wiley & Sons Inc; 2006. p. 959–63.

4. Park MJ, Paul Mulye T, Adams SH, et al. The health status of young adults in the United States. J Adolesc Health 2006;39:305–17.

5. Stutts JC, Wilkins JW, Scott Osberg J, et al. Driver risk factors for sleep-related crashes. Accid Anal Prev 2003;35:321–31.

6. Carskadon MA, Dement WC. Normal human sleep: an overview. In: Kryger MH, Roth T, Dement WC, editors. Principles and practice of sleep medicine. 4th edition. Philadelphia: Elsevier Saunders; 2005. p. 13–23.

7. Williams RL, Karacan I, Hursch CJ. EEG of human sleep: clinical applications. New York: John Wiley & Sons; 1974.

8. Ginsberg J, Gapen M. Academic worry as a predictor of sleep disturbance in college students. J Young Invest 2008;14. Available at: http://www.jyi.org/research/re.php?id=708. Accessed August 10, 2008.

9. National Sleep Foundation. Adolescent sleep needs and patterns: research report and resource guide. Washington, DC: National Sleep Foundation; 2000.

10. Bixler EO, Vgontzas AN, Lin HM, et al. Excessive daytime sleepiness in a general population sample: the role of sleep apnea, age, obesity, diabetes, and depression. J Clin Endocrinol Metab 2005;90:4510–5.

11. Millman RP, Working Group on Sleepiness in Adolescents/Young Adults, AAP Committee on Adolescence. Excessive sleepiness in adolescents and young adults: causes, consequences, and treatment strategies. Pediatrics 2005;115:1774–86.

12. Vela-Bueno A, Fernández-Mendoza J, Olavarrieta-Bernardino S, et al. Sleep and behavioural correlates of napping among young adults: a survey of first year university students in Madrid. J Am Coll Health 2008;57:150–8.

13. Johns MW. A new method for measuring daytime sleepiness: the Epworth sleepiness scale. Sleep 1991;14:540–5.

14. Moo-Estrella J, Pérez-Benítez H, Solís-Rodríguez F, et al. Evaluation of depressive symptoms and sleep alterations in college students. Arch Med Res 2005; 36:393–8.

15. American Academy of Sleep Medicine. The international classification of sleep disorders: diagnostic & coding manual, ICDS-2. 2nd edition. Westchester (IL): American Academy of Sleep Medicine; 2005.

16. Partinen M, Hublin C. Epidemiology of sleep disorders. In: Kryger MH, Roth T, Dement WC, editors. Principles and practice of sleep medicine. 4th edition. Philadelphia: Elsevier Saunders; 2005. p. 626–47.

17. Wittmann M, Dinich J, Merrow M, et al. Social jetlag: misalignment of biological and social time. Chronobiol Int 2006;23:497–509.

18. Lima PF, Medeiros AL, Araujo JF. Sleep-wake pattern of medical students: early versus late class starting time. Braz J Med Biol Res 2002;35:1373–7.

19. Buboltz WC Jr, Brown F, Soper B. Sleep habits and patterns of college students: a preliminary study. J Am Coll Health 2001;50:131–5.

20. Valdez P, Ramirez C, Garcia A. Delaying and extending sleep during weekends: sleep recovery or circadian effect? Chronobiol Int 1996;13:191–8.

21. Lack LC. Delayed sleep and sleep loss in university students. J Am Coll Health 1986;35:105–10.

22. Ferber R, Boyle MP. Delayed sleep phase syndrome versus motivated sleep phase delay. Sleep Research 1983;12:329.

23. Schrader H, Bovim G, Sand T. The prevalence of delayed and advanced sleep phase syndromes. J Sleep Res 1993;2:51–5.

24. Manber R, Bootzin RR, Acebo C, et al. The effects of regularizing sleep-wake schedules on daytime sleepiness. Sleep 1996;19:432–41.

25. Medeiros ALD, Mendes DBF, Lima PF, et al. The relationship between sleep-wake cycle and academic performance in medical students. Biol Rhythm Res 2001;32:263–70.

26. Ban DJ, Lee TJ. Sleep duration, subjective sleep disturbances and associated factors among university students in Korea. J Korean Med Sci 2001;16: 475–80.

27. Yang CM, Wu CH, Hsieh MH, et al. Coping with sleep disturbances among young adults: a survey of first-year college students in Taiwan. Behav Med 2003;29:133–8.

28. Tsai LL, Li SP. Sleep patterns in college students: gender and grade differences. J Psychosom Res 2004;56:231–7.

29. Steptoe A, Peacey V, Wardle J. Sleep duration and health in young adults. Arch Intern Med 2006;166: 1689–92.

30. Vela-Bueno A, Fernández-Mendoza J, Olavarrieta-Bernardino S, et al. Perceived sleep debt: cognitive, emotional and behavioral correlates in young adults. Sleep 2007;30:A141–2.

31. Dinges DF, Orne MT, Whitehouse WG, et al. Temporal placement of nap for alertness: contributions of circadian phase and prior wakefulness. Sleep 1987;10:313–29.

32. Dinges DF. Adult napping and its effects on ability to function. In: Stampi C, editor. Why we nap: evolution, chronobiology and functions of polyphasic and ultra-short sleep. Boston: Birkhaüser; 1992. p. 118–34.

33. Pilcher JJ, Kristin RM, Carrigan RD. The prevalence of daytime napping and its relationship to nighttime sleep. Behav Med 2001;27:71–6.

34. Taub JM. The sleep–wakefulness cycle in Mexican adults. J Cross Cult Psychol 1971;2:353–62.

35. Valencia-Flores M, Castaño VA, Campos RM, et al. The siesta culture concept is not supported by the sleep habits of urban Mexican students. J Sleep Res 1998;7:21–9.

36. Thorleifsdottir B, Björnsson JK, Benediktsdottir B, et al. Sleep and sleep habits from childhood to young adulthood over a 10-year period. J Psychosom Res 2002;53:529–37.

37. Takahashi M. The role of prescribed napping in sleep medicine. Sleep Med Rev 2003;7:227–35.

38. Brooks A, Lack L. Naps. In: Kushida CA, editor. Sleep deprivation: clinical issues, pharmacology and sleep loss effects. New York: Marcel Dekker; 2005. p. 457–74.

39. Takahashi M, Kaida K. Napping. In: Lee-Chiong T, editor. Sleep: a comprehensive handbook. Hoboken (NJ): John Wiley & Sons Inc.; 2006. p. 197–201.

40. Milner CE, Fogel SM, Cote KA. Habitual napping moderates motor performance improvements following a short daytime nap. Biol Psychol 2003; 73:141–56.

41. Lahl O, Wispel C, Willigens B, et al. An ultra short episode of sleep is sufficient to promote declarative memory performance. J Sleep Res 2008;17:3–10.

42. Tucker MA, Fishbein W. Enhancement of declarative memory performance following a daytime nap is contingent on strength of initial task acquisition. Sleep 2008;31:197–203.

43. Vgontzas AN, Pejovic S, Zoumakis E, et al. Daytime napping after a night of sleep loss decreases sleepiness, improves performance, and causes beneficial changes in cortisol and interleukin-6 secretion. Am J Physiol Endocrinol Metab 2007;292:253–61.

44. Trockel MT, Barnes MD, Egget DL. Health-related variables and academic performance among first-year college students: implications for sleep and other behaviors. J Am Coll Health 2000;49: 125–31.

45. Kelly WE, Kelly KE, Clanton RC. The relationship between sleep length and grade-point average among college students. Coll Stud J 2001;35:84–6.

Observation of the Natural Evolution of Insomnia in the American General Population Cohort

Maurice M. Ohayon, MD, DSc, PhD[a,b,*]

KEYWORDS

- Epidemiology • Insomnia • Depression • Anxiety
- Longitudinal data • Organic diseases • Pain

Insomnia symptoms are the most frequent sleep disturbances, affecting about one third of the general population.[1] Factors associated with insomnia symptoms are numerous; mental disorders and organic diseases are among the most frequently observed associations. Nonetheless, epidemiologic studies examining these associations remain uncommon, partly because of the complexity of assessing mental disorders in the general population and the costs involved in doing lengthy interviews. Longitudinal studies examining the evolution of insomnia symptoms are nearly nonexistent and are limited in the associations studied. This article briefly reviews the existing studies that have examined the associations between insomnia and mental disorders along with consequences of insomnia. New data on a longitudinal study performed at the Stanford Sleep Epidemiology Research Center are presented also.

ASSOCIATION BETWEEN MENTAL DISORDERS AND INSOMNIA

Cross-sectional studies have shown that 40% to 60% of subjects who have insomnia exhibit symptoms of depression.[2–5] Clinical depression was observed in 10% to 25% of insomnia cases.[6–12] Anxiety is more common: 20% to 30% of subjects who had insomnia also had anxiety disorders.[6–8,11,12]

The diagnostic distribution of subjects who have insomnia is presented in **Fig. 1**. Mental disorders are observed in 30% to 40% of persons who have insomnia complaints. Sleep-related breathing disorders such as obstructive sleep apnea syndrome or hypoventilation account for 5% to 9% of insomnia complaints.[1,13,14] Periodic limb movement disorders and/or restless legs syndrome are found in about 15% of individuals who have insomnia complaints.[1,13,15,16] Medical or neurologic conditions are observed in 4% to 11% of insomnia complaints.[1,13,14] Poor sleep hygiene or environmental factors account for about 10% of insomnia complaints, and 3% to 7% of insomnia complaints are substance induced.[1] Multiple associated conditions can be observed in as many as 30% of individuals who have insomnia complaints.[17]

Several cross-sectional studies have highlighted the association between insomnia, depression, and anxiety. Little, however, is known about

The author was supported by National Institutes of Health grant R01NS044199, by the Arrillaga Foundation, and the Bing Foundation.

[a] Department of Psychiatry and Behavioral Sciences, School of Medicine, Stanford University, 401 Quarry Road, Stanford, CA 94305, USA
[b] Stanford Sleep Epidemiology Research Center (SSERC), School of Medicine, Stanford University, 3430 W. Bayshore Road, Palo Alto, CA 94303, USA
* Stanford Sleep Epidemiology Research Centre (SSERC), School of Medicine, Stanford University, 3430 W. Bayshore Road, Palo Alto, CA 94303, USA.
E-mail address: mohayon@stanford.edu

Sleep Med Clin 4 (2009) 87–92
doi:10.1016/j.jsmc.2008.12.002

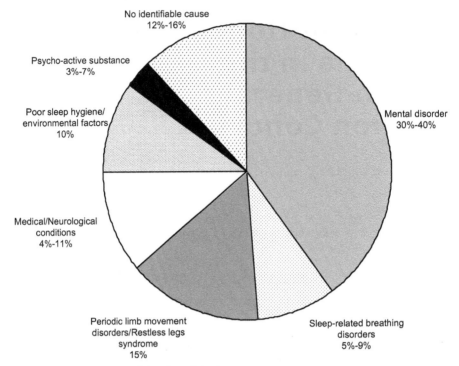

Fig. 1. Distribution of insomnia complaints by etiologic causes.

factors that may influence this relationship. Consequently, a better control over other predictors of mental disorders such as obesity or chronic pain might offer a clearer picture of the association between mental disorder and insomnia.

From longitudinal studies, it is known that insomnia at point 1 predicts depression at point 2.[18–22] Furthermore, the persistence of insomnia (present in both evaluations) is a stronger predictor of depression at point 2.[19,21,23]

Most longitudinal studies have analyzed the association of insomnia and mental disorders as a unidimensional phenomenon, but multidimensional models would be more appropriate. It is not yet known what extent insomnia is a precursor rather than a cause of mental disorder.

CONSEQUENCES OF INSOMNIA

The consequences of insomnia can manifest at several levels:

- Development of a medical condition
- Development of a mental disorder
- Repercussions on daytime functioning
- Road, work, and domestic accidents

Development of a Medical Condition

Several studies have attempted to determine whether insomnia might be responsible for cardiovascular accidents, but the results are inconclusive. One study found that individuals who had insomnia had a 3.1 relative risk of experiencing a cardiovascular accident,[24] but other studies found no causality between insomnia and the risk of developing a cardiovascular disease, and another study found a greater likelihood of developing insomnia after a cardiovascular accident.[25]

Development of a Mental Disorder

A study[7] examining the time sequence between insomnia and mood and anxiety disorders reported that insomnia was present in 70% of subjects who had mood disorders and that insomnia preceded the manifestation of the mood disorders in nearly half of cases (**Fig. 2**A). Insomnia was found in one third of the subjects who had anxiety disorders. Insomnia symptoms preceded the anxiety disorders in about one fifth of the cases (**Fig. 2**B).

Repercussions on Daytime Functioning

Daytime functioning is affected in 20% to 60% of individuals who have insomnia.[10,11,26–28] Individuals who poorly sleep at least 3 nights per week, who are dissatisfied with their sleep, who are unrested upon awakening, and who have hyperarousal in bed are the most likely to have repercussions on daytime functioning.[10,11]

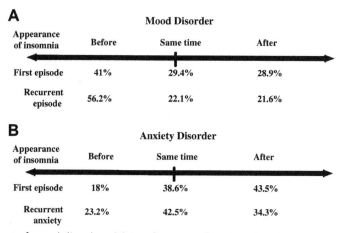

Fig. 2. (*A*) Development of mood disorders. (*B*) Development of anxiety disorders.

Road, Occupational, and Domestic Accidents

Road accidents are two to three times more frequent in drivers who are dissatisfied with their sleep.[9,10] Road accidents also are more frequent in short sleepers (< 5 hours).[29,30] In elderly persons, insomnia was associated with an increased risk of hip fracture[31] and falls.[32,33] Another study found a relative risk of 1.9 for fatal occupational accidents in individuals who had difficulty in sleeping.[34]

ASSOCIATIONS BETWEEN PAIN, MENTAL DISORDERS, ORGANIC DISEASES, AND INSOMNIA SYMPTOMS

The Venn's diagram in **Fig. 3** shows the interaction between insomnia symptoms, mental disorders, organic diseases, and dyssomnia diagnoses (insomnia disorder, obstructive sleep apnea,

restless legs syndrome, circadian rhythm disorders, and hypersomnia/narcolepsy) (M. Ohayon, personal data on the European population, 2007). As seen, insomnia symptoms rarely occur alone. In half of the cases a concurrent organic disease is observed; in a third of the cases a mental disorder is present; and organic disease and mental disorder are present in 1 of 10 cases.

In nearly 70% of cases, mental disorders are concomitant with organic diseases and/or other dyssomnias. More than 50% of organic diseases are accompanied by mental disorders and/or other dyssomnias.

The Venn's diagram in **Fig. 4** shows the associations between chronic pain, mental disorders, organic diseases, and insomnia symptoms in the American general population (M. Ohayon, personal data, 2007). Insomnia symptoms are associated with chronic pain in up to 66.8% of cases. Similarly, 72% of subjects who have mental

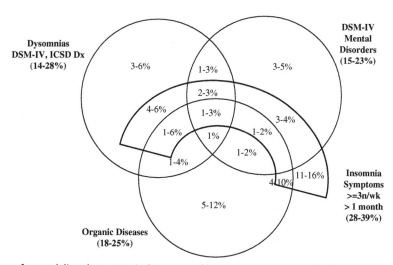

Fig. 3. Association of mental disorders, organic diseases, and insomnia symptoms in the European general population.

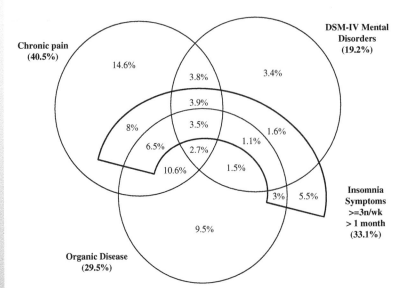

Fig. 4. Association of chronic pain, mental disorders, organic diseases, and insomnia symptoms in the American general population.

disorders and 79% of subjects who have organic disease also have chronic pain.

EVOLUTION OF INSOMNIA AND MENTAL DISORDERS

A longitudinal study of a representative sample of the California general population was undertaken in 2005 and 2006 at the Stanford Sleep Epidemiology Research Center. The baseline sample included 3249 adults from the general population interviewed between 2002 and 2003. At the end of the interview, they were asked if they were willing to be interviewed again in the future; 2729 agreed to be part of the longitudinal survey.

The follow-up was done 3 years after the initial interview. From the baseline sample, 1957 individuals were reached. Among participants lost to follow-up, 17 had died; 41 were seriously ill or hospitalized; 132 refused to participate, 203 telephone numbers had been assigned to a new household; and 379 telephone numbers had been disconnected.

Evolution of Insomnia

At baseline, 42.1% of the 1957 individuals who participated in the follow-up had insomnia symptoms at least 3 nights per week for at least 1 month. Three years later, 72.2% of them still had insomnia symptoms. Among those who did not have insomnia symptoms at baseline, 15.5% developed insomnia symptoms (**Fig. 5**).

The author examined whether pre-existing chronic pain (pain lasting for at least 3 months) and mental disorders (without insomnia symptoms) were predictors for the development of

insomnia. After adjusting for age, gender, and race, the investigators found that individuals who had a major depressive disorder had a relative risk of 3.8 of developing insomnia at 3-year follow-up. The relative risk of developing insomnia was 2.6 among individuals who had anxiety disorder and 1.8 among individuals who had chronic pain.

The author also examined whether insomnia symptoms were predictors for the development of chronic pain and mental disorders. Subjects who had insomnia symptoms but who did not have a major depressive disorder at baseline had a relative risk of 2.1 of developing a major depressive disorder at 3-year follow-up. Subjects who had insomnia symptoms but who did not have anxiety disorder at baseline had a relative risk of

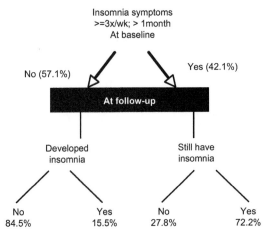

Fig. 5. Evolution of insomnia symptoms in the California sample.

1.9 of developing an anxiety disorder at 3-year follow-up. The presence of insomnia at baseline was not associated significantly with chronic pain at 3-year follow-up.

SUMMARY

Existing cross-sectional epidemiologic studies tend to examine associations between insomnia and mental disorders only in a bi-dimensional way. Many other factors related to both insomnia and mental disorders might have confounding effects on this association. One of the possible consequences would be an amplification effect on odds ratios when no control is exerted on possible confounding variables. The two Venn's diagrams show that insomnia symptoms and mental disorders often are associated also with several organic diseases and chronic pain.

In the reported longitudinal study, the author has demonstrated that insomnia, psychiatric disorders, organic diseases, and pain are closely inter-related. Major depressive disorder at baseline was the strongest predictor of developing insomnia. Insomnia at baseline was associated with a three-fold increased risk of developing a major depressive disorder and anxiety at 3-year follow-up. Further analyses of the effects of confounding variables will offer a clearer picture on how insomnia is closely related to the development of a psychiatric disorder.

REFERENCES

1. Ohayon MM. Epidemiology of insomnia: what we know and what we still need to learn. Sleep Med Rev 2002;6:97–111.
2. Foley DJ, Monjan AA, Brown SL, et al. Sleep complaints among elderly persons: an epidemiologic study of three communities. Sleep 1995;18:425–32.
3. Henderson S, Jorm AF, Scott LR, et al. Insomnia in the elderly: its prevalence and correlates in the general population. Med J Aust 1995;162:22–4.
4. Mellinger GD, Balter MB, Uhlenhuth EH. Insomnia and its treatment: prevalence and correlates. Arch Gen Psychiatry 1985;42:225–32.
5. Ohayon MM, Caulet M, Lemoine P. Comorbidity of mental and insomnia disorders in the general population. Compr Psychiatry 1998;39:185–97.
6. Maggi S, Langlois JA, Minicuci N, et al. Sleep complaints in community-dwelling older persons: prevalence, associated factors, and reported causes. J Am Geriatr Soc 1998;46:161–8.
7. Ohayon MM, Roth T. Place of chronic insomnia in the course of depressive and anxiety disorders. J Psychiatr Res 2003;37:9–15.
8. Ohayon MM, Shapiro CM, Kennedy SH. Differentiating DSM-IV anxiety and depressive disorders in the general population: comorbidity and treatment consequences. Can J Psychiatry 2000;45:166–72.
9. Ohayon MM, Smirne S. Prevalence and consequences of insomnia disorders in the general population of Italy. Sleep Med 2002;3:115–20.
10. Ohayon MM, Roth T. What are the contributing factors for insomnia in the general population? J Psychosom Res 2001;51:745–55.
11. Ohayon MM. Prevalence of DSM-IV diagnostic criteria of insomnia: distinguishing between insomnia related to mental disorders from sleep disorders. J Psychiatr Res 1997;31:333–46.
12. Taylor DJ, Lichstein KL, Durrence HH, et al. Epidemiology of insomnia, depression, and anxiety. Sleep 2005;28:1457–64.
13. Buysse DJ, Reynold CF, Hauri P, et al. Diagnostic concordance for DSM-IV disorders: a report from the APA/NIMH DSM-IV field trial. Am J Psychiatry 1994;151:1351–60.
14. Jacobs EA, Reynolds CF 3rd, Kupfer DJ, et al. The role of polysomnography in the differential diagnosis of chronic insomnia. Am J Psychiatry 1988;145:346–9.
15. Edinger JD, Fins AI, Goeke JM, et al. The empirical identification of insomnia subtypes: a cluster analytic approach. Sleep 1996;19:398–411.
16. Ohayon MM, Roth T. Prevalence of restless legs syndrome and periodic limb movement disorder in the general population. J Psychosom Res 2002;53:547–54.
17. Ohayon MM. Interlacing sleep, pain, mental disorders and organic diseases. J Psychiatr Res 2006;40:677–9.
18. Breslau N, Roth T, Rosenthal L, et al. Sleep disturbance and psychiatric disorders: a longitudinal epidemiological study of young adults. Biol Psychiatry 1996;39:411–8.
19. Ford DE, Kamerow DB. Epidemiologic study of sleep disturbances and psychiatric disorders. An opportunity for prevention? JAMA 1989;262:1479–84.
20. Jansson M, Linton SJ. The development of insomnia within the first year: a focus on worry. Br J Health Psychol 2006;11(Pt 3):501–11.
21. Roberts RE, Shema SJ, Kaplan GA, et al. Sleep complaints and depression in an aging cohort: a prospective perspective. Am J Psychiatry 2000;157:81–8.
22. Weissman MM, Greenwald S, Niño-Murcia G, et al. The morbidity of insomnia uncomplicated by psychiatric disorders. Gen Hosp Psychiatry 1997;19:245–50.
23. Perlis ML, Smith LJ, Lyness JM, et al. Insomnia as a risk factor for onset of depression in the elderly. Behav Sleep Med 2006;4:104–13.
24. Mallon L, Broman JE, Hetta J. Sleep complaints predict coronary artery disease mortality in males: a

12-year follow-up study of a middle-aged Swedish population. J Intern Med 2002;251:207–16.

25. Foley DJ, Monjan A, Simonsick EM, et al. Incidence and remission of insomnia among elderly adults: an epidemiologic study of 6,800 persons over three years. Sleep 1999;22(Suppl 2):S366–72.

26. Hetta J, Broman JE, Mallon L. Evaluation of severe insomnia in the general population—implications for the management of insomnia: insomnia, quality of life and healthcare consumption in Sweden. J Psychopharmacol 1999;13(4 Suppl 1):S35–6.

27. Hoffmann G. Evaluation of severe insomnia in the general population—implications for the management of insomnia: focus on results from Belgium. J Psychopharmacol 1999;13(4 Suppl 1):S31–2.

28. Leger D, Guilleminault C, Dreyfus JP, et al. Prevalence of insomnia in a survey of 12,778 adults in France. J Sleep Res 2000;9:35–42.

29. Connor J, Norton R, Ameratunga S, et al. Driver sleepiness and risk of serious injury to car occupants: population based case control study. BMJ 2002;324:1125.

30. McCartt AT, Ribner SA, Pack AI, et al. The scope and nature of the drowsy driving problem in New York State. Accid Anal Prev 1996;28:511–7.

31. Fitzpatrick P, Kirke PN, Daly L, et al. Predictors of first hip fracture and mortality post fracture in older women. Ir J Med Sci 2001;170:49–53.

32. Brassington GS, King AC, Bliwise DL. Sleep problems as a risk factor for falls in a sample of community-dwelling adults aged 64–99 years. J Am Geriatr Soc 2000;48:1234–40.

33. Méndez Rubio JI, Zunzunegui MV, Béland F, et al. [The prevalence of and factors associated with falls in older persons living in the community]. Med Clin (Barc) 1997;108:128–32 [in Spanish].

34. Akerstedt T, Fredlund P, Gillberg M, et al. A prospective study of fatal occupational accidents—relationship to sleeping difficulties and occupational factors. J Sleep Res 2002;11:69–71.

Index

Note: Page numbers of article titles are in **boldface** type.

Sleep Med Clin 4 (2009) 93–97
doi:10.1016/S1556-407X(09)00030-7
1556-407X/09/$ – see front matter

Moving?

Make sure your subscription moves with you!

To notify us of your new address, find your **Clinics Account Number** (located on your mailing label above your name), and contact customer service at:

E-mail: elspcs@elsevier.com

800-654-2452 (subscribers in the U.S. & Canada)
314-453-7041 (subscribers outside of the U.S. & Canada)

Fax number: 314-523-5170

Elsevier Periodicals Customer Service
11830 Westline Industrial Drive
St. Louis, MO 63146

*To ensure uninterrupted delivery of your subscription, please notify us at least 4 weeks in advance of move.

Printed and bound by CPI Group (UK) Ltd, Croydon, CR0 4YY

03/10/2024

01040360-0016